AF762807

P. Buchmann W. Brühlmann (Eds.)

# Investigation of Anorectal Functional Disorders

With Special Emphasis on Defaecography

With 130 Figures, Some in Colour,
and 38 Tables

Springer-Verlag
Berlin Heidelberg New York London Paris
Tokyo Hong Kong Barcelona Budapest

Professor Dr. Peter Buchmann
Chirurgische Klinik, Stadtspital Waid
Tièchestrasse 99, 8037 Zürich, Switzerland

Professor Dr. Werner Brühlmann
Institut für Röntgendiagnostik
Stadtspital Triemli
Birmensdorferstrasse 497, 8063 Zürich, Switzerland

ISBN-13:978-3-642-77404-1 e-ISBN-13:978-3-642-77402-7
DOI: 10.1007/978-3-642-77402-7

Library of Congress Cataloging-in-Publication Data
Investigation of anorectal functional disorders: with special emphasis on defaecography/P. Buchmann, W. Brühlmann, eds. P.cm.
Includes bibliographical references and index.
ISBN-13:978-3-642-77404-1
1. Defecation disorders – Diagnosis – Congresses. 2. Anorectal function tests – Congresses. 3. Defecography – Congresses.
I. Buchmann, P. (Peter) II. Brühlmann, W. (Werner)
RC866.D43I59 1993 616.3'5 – dc20 92-26472

This work is subject to copyright. All rights are reserved, whether the whole or part of the material is concerned, specifically the rights of translation, reprinting, reuse of illustrations, recitation, broadcasting, reproduction on microfilm or in any other way, and storage in data banks. Duplication of this publication or parts thereof is permitted only under the provisions of the German Copyright Law of September 9, 1965, in its current version, and permission for use must always be obtained from Springer-Verlag. Violations are liable for prosecution under the German Copyright Law.

© Springer-Verlag Berlin Heidelberg 1993
Softcover reprint of the hardcover 1st edition 1983

The use of general descriptive names, registered names, trademarks, etc. in this publication does not imply, even in the absence of a specific statement, that such names are exempt from the relevant protective laws and regulations and therefore free for general use.

Product liability: The publishers cannot guarantee the accuracy of any information about dosage and application contained in this book. In every individual case the user must check such information by consulting the relevant literature.

Typesetting: Best-set Typesetter Ltd., Hong Kong
24/3130-5 4 3 2 1 0 – Printed on acid-free paper

# Preface

Medical examination of the anus and lower rectum has a very long tradition. The first instrument utilized was the doctor's finger, and digital examination is still the most important step after a precise case history. Endoscopy, first with a short tube, then with a rigid sigmoidoscope, enabled physicians to look inside the large intestine as far as 25 cm ab ano.

In 1919, Holzknecht introduced X-ray examination of the colon with contrast enema, but research concentrating on the physiology and pathophysiology of the anorectum and pelvic floor did not start until the second half of this century.

Many of the newly developed investigations have the disadvantage of influencing their own result (e.g. balloon size in manometry) or interfering with physiology (e.g. bowel preparation for endoscopy or double-contrast examination). Defaecography and scintigraphy are designed to investigate bowel motility. Defaecography in particular demonstrates the phase of rectal emptying, yet the value and range of indications for this new method have not been clearly defined. We therefore organized a workshop, held in May 1991, the results of which are presented in this book. We hope, that this volume will help the physician in selecting the appropriate investigations and in performing and interpreting them.

We warmly thank the firms that supported our workshop: Auto Suture (Swiss) AG, Hoeri; Blendax-Richardson AG, Geneva; Eli Lilly S.A., Geneva; Hofmann-La Roche, Basel; Johnson & Johnson AG, Spreitenbach; Kali-Duphar Pharma AG, Bern; Kodak, Lausanne; Medichemie AG, Ettlingen; Phardi AG, Basel; Philips Medical Systems AG, Zürich; Sandoz-Wander Pharma AG, Bern; Schering (Swiss) AG, Schlieren; Searle S.A., Lausanne.

Our thanks go to all the contributors, to Mrs. Dovian for the workshop administration, to Mrs. Flückiger for the manuscript management and, last but not least, to Springer-Verlag Heidelberg for publishing the book.

Zürich, autumn 1992

W. Brühlmann
P. Buchmann

# Contents

# List of Senior Authors

Buchmann, Peter, Prof. Dr. med.
Chirurgische Klinik, Stadtspital Waid
Tièchestrasse 99, 8037 Zürich, Switzerland

Brühlmann, Werner, Prof. Dr. med.
Institut für Röntgendiagnostik, Stadtspital Triemli
Birmensdorferstrasse 497, 8063 Zürich, Switzerland

Erckenbrecht, J.F., Prof. Dr. med.
Medizinische Klinik, Krankenanstalten
"Florence Nightingale", Kreuzbergstrasse 79
W-4000 Düsseldorf 31 (Kaiserswerth), FRG

Geile, Dorothee, Dr. med.
Einsteinstrasse 127, W-8000 München 80, FRG

Goei, Reginald, Dr. med.
Department of Radiology, De Wever Hospital
PO Box 4446, 6401 CX Heerlen, The Netherlands

Hauck, Reiner, Dr. med.
Maximilianstrasse 14, W-8000 München 22, FRG

Hildebrandt, U., PD Dr. med.
Chirurgische Klinik, Universitätskliniken des Saarlandes
W-6650 Homburg/Saar, FRG

Hirsig, Johannes, Dr. med.
FMH für Kinderchirurgie
Zürichstrasse 63, 8424 Embrach, Switzerland

Kamm, Michael A., Dr. med.
St. Mark's Hospital, City Road
London EC1V 2PS, United Kingdom

Kuijpers, H.C., Dr. med.
Allgemene Chirurgie, Academisch Ziekenhuis Nijmegen
Geert Grooteplein 14, Postbus 9101
6500 HB Nijmegen, The Netherlands

Mahieu, P.H.G., Dr. med.
Department of Radiology UCL
Surgical Institute of Brussels
59, Square Marie-Louise, 1040 Brussels, Belgium

Marti, M.-C., Prof. Dr. med.
Hôpital Cantonal Universitaire, 24, rue Michelin-du-Crest
1211 Genève 4, Switzerland

Rühl, A., Dr.
Medizinische Klinik, Krankenanstalten
"Florence Nightingale", Kreuzbergstrasse 79
W-4000 Düsseldorf 31 (Kaiserswerth), FRG

Stuckmann, G., Dr. med.
Röntgendiagnostik, Kantonsspital
Brauerstrasse 15, 8401 Winterthur, Switzerland

# 1 Physiology and Pathophysiology of Defaecation

M.A. Kamm

The process of defaecation is complex and depends on the integration of neurological information from the brain, spinal cord, pelvic floor and colon itself. Once this information has been processed the act of defaecation relies on intact colonic and pelvic floor function. Other factors which contribute to this process include the colonic contents (bile acids, fatty acids, water and fibre content), gender, age, personality and hormonal status.

## 1.1 Extrinsic Control of Colonic Motor Function

Our knowledge about the cerebral control of large bowel function remains rudimentary, yet it is likely that many disorders of defaecation derive from an abnormality of this regulation. Recent animal studies have revealed specific cerebral control sites and neurotransmitters [1]. The hypothalamus directly affects colonic activity: the intracerebroventricular injection of thyrotropin-releasing hormone produces an increase in motility [2]. Experimental work in animals has also demonstrated an important central role of thyrotropin-releasing hormone and corticotropin-releasing hormone in influencing gastrointestinal transit and faecal output. Changes in colonic motility associated with stress can be shown to be related to intracerebral release of corticotropin-releasing hormone [3]. Opioids also influence colonic activity, some of them by their central action in the brain or spinal cord [4, 5]. Undoubtedly other neurotransmitters of importance will emerge.

It is possible that disturbances of colonic motility and defaecation in some patients derive from abnormal cerebral control. Evidence in support of this comes from the disturbed colonic function and constipation observed after a cerebrovascular accident, including subarachnoid haemorrhage, although the changes may be due in part to altered peripheral autonomic function and are usually not permanent. Colonic transit can be delayed after an anterior or posterior pontine lesion [6]. In multiple sclerosis, constipation affects more than 40% of patients [7], although the exact relationship of cerebral or spinal plaques to altered motility remains to be determined.

Perhaps the most interesting association is that between psychological disturbance and altered defaecation. Normal individuals can slow their colonic transit and decrease their defaecation frequency if given a financial incentive, illustrating the powerful link between brain and bowel [8]. The opposite is also true – stress is a well-known cause of increased colonic transit and diarrhoea. Stress, anxiety and depression are all increased in prevalence in hospital patients with the irritable bowel syndrome, and are thought to have an aetiological role, although recent community-based studies have cast doubt on this by revealing that patients with irritable bowel syndrome in the community have a normal psychological profile [9, 10].

Could personality factors or disturbed psychology cause severe constipation? Young women with severe idiopathic constipation have a high prevalence of adverse early life events [11] and disturbed psychological profile [12]; in some of these patients biofeedback conditioning aimed at relaxing the pelvic floor relieves the constipation [13], although the effect may be via general relaxation and therefore altered cerebral regulation. It is tempting to speculate that a central neurotransmitter disturbance could cause both an altered psychological state and decreased colonic motility. Alternative explanations include changed autonomic regulation due to central factors, or a centrally mediated change in the circulating hormones which regulate motility.

An intact spinal cord is also important in maintaining normal colonic function. Constipation is extremely common in paraplegics, and colonic compliance is markedly decreased after a complete thoracic spinal cord lesion. Constipation caused by spinal trauma is presumably due to denervation of the parasympathetic supply to the left colon; such patients show left colonic delay and may show morphological changes of the myenteric plexus similar to those seen in patients with idiopathic constipation [14]. Onuf's nucleus in the sacral cord supplies the innervation to the somatic pelvic floor muscles and coordinates integrated pelvic floor muscle activity during defaecation and micturition.

The pelvic sacral parasympathetic nerves provide a motor drive to the left colon. Damage to these nerves will also cause intractable constipation [15].

## 1.2 Colonic Motility

The *patterns* of colonic, rectal and anal sphincter motility are largely determined by neural circuits within the bowel wall. In this respect the large bowel is no different to the more proximal gastrointestinal tract. Although dependent to some extent on extrinsic innervation to maintain their integrity, the intrinsic nerves can autonomously regulate colonic contractions and movement. The major neural network responsible for the regulation of colonic motor activity, the myenteric plexus, is situated between the circular and longitudinal smooth muscle layers of the bowel wall. It regulates the coordinated contractile activity of these two muscle layers, but is also dependent on receiving sensory information from luminal receptors and the

submucosal plexus. The physical and chemical properties of the colonic contents influence colonic motor activity via these neural networks.
The patterns of colonic motor activity have been well characterised in recent years [16]. Most of the time the colon is involved in segmenting activity which is responsible for mixing the colonic contents and bringing them into contact with the mucosa so that water and nutrients can be absorbed. These segmenting contractions are not coordinated between different colonic regions. The existence of a higher pressure segmenting zone in the sigmoid or at the rectosigmoid junction is controversial.
Several times during 24 h a high pressure peristaltic wave, or mass movement, transports colonic contents along the colon. These colonic movements were first observed by Cannon [17] and Holzknecht in radiological studies of animals in the earliest part of this century. The pressure in these peristaltic waves may be as high as 200 mmHg, and recent studies using radioisotopes have confirmed that they are the major motor event causing the transport of colonic contents [18].

## 1.3 The Colon During Defaecation

Studies in dogs, in which strain gauges were sewn on to the colonic serosa, have shown that some of these mass movements, which may start at almost any point in the colon, progress only partly along the length of the large bowel. Some mass movements in the dog progressed far enough along the colon to be associated with defaecation and cause colonic emptying [19].
Does the same process occur in humans? It has been difficult to record motility changes in man using pressure-measuring devices during spontaneous defaecation. However, defaecation can be induced using a predictable motor stimulant such as bisacodyl. Such studies have demonstrated that the pattern of colonic motility is similar in man. Colonic peristalsis can be induced at any point along the colon, producing peristaltic waves that traverse the length of the colon, causing defaecation with colonic emptying [20]. This activity is associated with rectal contraction, although the amplitude of the activity is less in the rectum than in the more proximal large bowel. Anal sphincter relaxation, due to relaxation of the smooth muscle internal anal sphincter, occurs early in this process, well before the peristaltic wave reaches the rectum [18] (Fig. 1.1). Anal relaxation therefore appears to be mediated by the intramural nerves well in advance of the peristaltic wave, in a similar manner to the lower oesophageal sphincter relaxation associated with swallowing. Schang and Devroede have shown that descending colonic and rectal contraction, associated with migrating electrical activity, leads to anal relaxation [21] (Fig. 1.2), although this anal relaxation did not occur as early as in other studies [18].
During defaecation a variable amount of the colon is emptied. Halls showed in 1965, using orally ingested radio-opaque markers in healthy subjects, that

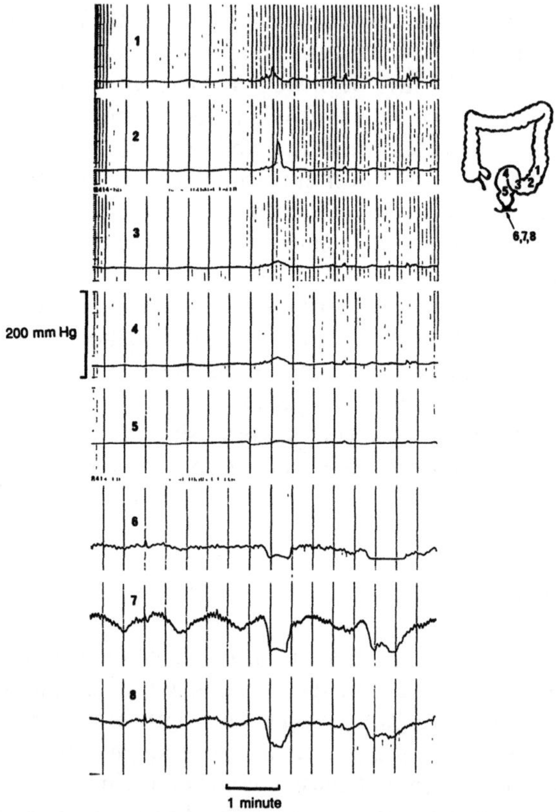


**Fig. 1.1.** Example of colonic peristalsis with rectal contraction and associated anal sphincter relaxation. In this example colonic activity was initiated by infusing bisacodyl solution into the descending colon. Simultaneous with colonic contraction there was movement and expulsion of previously instilled radio-isotope. See van der Sijp et al. [18].

the colon can empty from as much as the distal transverse colon to as little as just the rectum [22]. When defaecation is suppressed, retrograde movement of colonic contents occurs.

Abnormalities of colonic peristalsis appear to be the most important motor abnormality in patients with severe constipation. In patients with severe constipation and a colon of normal diameter, there is a reduction in the frequency and duration of colonic peristaltic waves [23]. They also appear not to progress as far along the large bowel. In diarrhoea-predominant irritable bowel patients there is an increase in the number of these peristaltic waves [24].

The coordination of colonic peristalsis depends on the integrity of the intrinsic neural networks. Many neurotransmitters appear to be involved in this process, but amongst the most important are vasoactive intestinal poly-

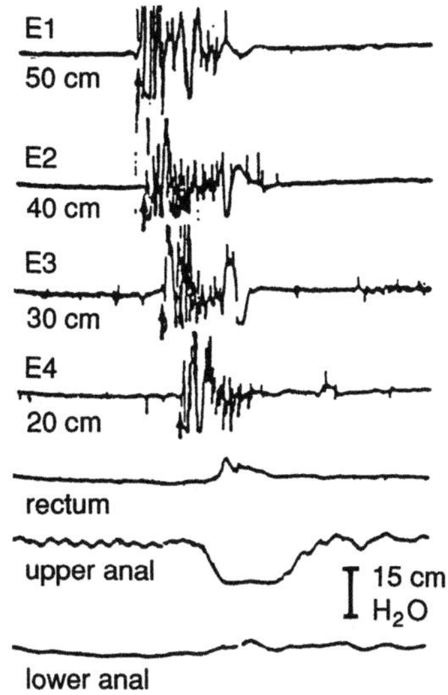


**Fig. 1.2.** Colonic peristalsis is associated with propagating spiking electrical activity. This electrical activity progresses distally, is associated with rectal contraction and leads to internal sphincter relaxation. (Schang and Devroede [21])

peptide (VIP), which mediates the descending relaxation component of peristalsis, and 5-hydroxytryptamine, present in regulatory interneurons. Abnormalities of these substances have been identified in the resected colon of patients with severe constipation, in particular a diminished concentration of VIP [25] and an elevated concentration of 5-hydroxytryptamine [26]. Morphological studies have also shown an abnormal appearance of neurons in the myenteric plexus of such patients [27].

The precise events that trigger the desire to defaecate or initiate defaecation are not known. For defaecation to occur, usually an individual senses an abdominal sensation of "fullness" or need to evacuate. On other occasions the colon may have already started to contract, a high pressure develops in the colon, and the subject experiences "urgency". In patients with the irritable bowel syndrome, sigmoid luminal pressures are surprisingly high, and certainly higher than normal [28]. Colonic contraction or urgency can be opposed by contraction of the striated sphincter muscles and pelvic floor, and this suppression results in retrograde colonic movement. Defaecation can also be voluntarily initiated when no desire to defaecate is present, by straining; under these circumstances the rise in intra-abdominal pressure together with the removal of cerebral inhibition stimulates the appropriate neural "programme" within the colon or rectum to initiate motor activity.

Factors which affect the frequency of defaecation are well recognised. Personality affects defaecation frequency – individuals who are more extrovert defaecate more often and have a higher stool output than introspective individuals [29]. An increase in dietary fibre causes increased stool output and bowel frequency; several mechanisms are involved, including an increase in colonic bacterial mass and a mechanical irritating effect on the epithelial surface [30]. Increasing the water load to the colon causes distension and peristalsis, as in small bowel infection with cholera. Inflammation and infection in the colon not only cause secretion but probably also stimulate colonic nerves. Rectal disease causes decreased colonic compliance and increased frequency and urgency, such as is seen in patients with radiation proctitis.

What role does the rectum play in defaecation? In most people the rectum is not a major site for faecal storage; the rectum is empty or contains only a small amount of stool in normal people most of the time. Studies of stimulated defaecation using bisacodyl suggest that the rectum can contract and is held as a rigid muscular tube through which colonic contents are squeezed. Alternatively, if there is some stool in the rectum, defaecation probably can be achieved by an alternative mechanism in which the subject strains; simultaneous with this, extrinsic nerves are activated to cause sphincter relaxation. The associated rise in intra-abdominal pressure, perhaps aided by rectal contraction, helps to empty the rectum.

## 1.4 The Pelvic Floor During Defaecation

During defaecation a particular sequence of events occurs at the level of the pelvic floor which allows rectal emptying. As the peristalsis approaches, the internal anal sphincter, which normally provides 85% of the resting anal tone, relaxes so that the anal pressure falls [18]. This internal anal sphincter relaxation is associated with cessation of its normal electrical slow wave activity [31]. The tonically active striated muscle external anal sphincter and puborectalis muscles are also inhibited, contributing to the fall in anal canal pressure (Fig. 1.3).

Associated with these changes in muscle activity, certain anatomical changes occur. Relaxation of the striated sphincter muscles and contraction of other parts of the levator plate cause straightening of the rectum so that it forms a less acute angle with the anal canal. The anal canal dilates as faecal material is passed.

### *1.4.1 Abnormalities of Pelvic Floor Function During Defaecation*

Does isolated rectal dysfunction lead to abnormal defaecation? Undoubtedly some patients with a solitary rectal ulcer, mucosal prolapse or full-thickness rectal prolapse have difficulty emptying their rectum for anatomical reasons. However, many such patients have a long-standing defaecatory disorder which preceded their anorectal disturbance, and these anatomical changes may be secondary. A rectocoele is thought to lead to poor rectal evacuation in some women, with the rectum failing to form a rigid muscular funnel; however, this anatomical variation is also seen in women who are asymptomatic [32, 33].

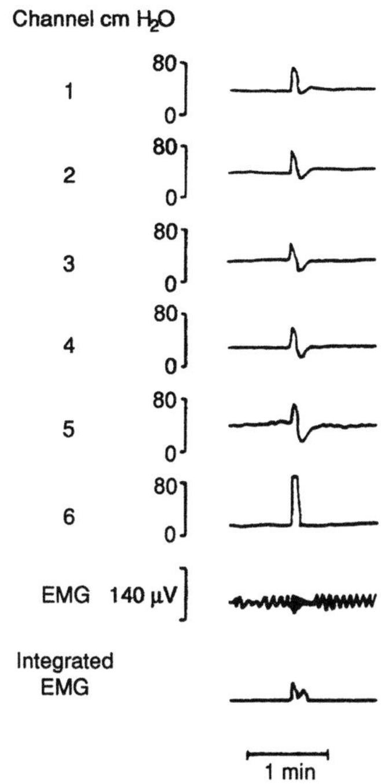


**Fig. 1.3.** Changes in anal canal pressure and smooth and striated anal muscle activity during straining. After an initial rise the anal canal pressure falls, and this is associated with loss of the internal anal sphincter electrical slow wave activity. The integrated electromyographic signal from the striated muscle external anal sphincter also falls. (Sun et al. [31])

Much interest has centred on patients with constipation who do not relax their pelvic floor striated muscles during defaecation straining. Patients with severe idiopathic constipation often inappropriately contract, rather than relax, their striated pelvic floor muscles [34]. This contraction of the puborectalis and external sphincter muscles has been postulated to cause an increase in anal canal pressure, thereby blocking rectal emptying. However, there is increasing evidence to suggest that this abnormal activity is a secondary learned phenomenon, and not primarily responsible for the constipation: the rectum is empty in most of these patients [35], suggesting a failure of colonic delivery to the distal bowel. Paralysis [36] or division of the striated muscles [37, 38] does not cure most patients of their symptoms. Paradoxical activity is not seen in all such patients, and is seen in patients with other conditions who are not constipated [39]. Lastly, the pattern of muscle activity observed in the anorectal laboratory may give a misleading impression since ambulatory electromyographic studies in constipated subjects thought to have inappropriate contraction during straining (in the laboratory) have shown that most relax their pelvic floor appropriately at home [40].

There is, however, evidence of abnormal rectal function in constipation. Rectal sensation is impaired in constipated patients who have a normal diameter rectum [41], and rectal motor function is also likely to be impaired.

Lastly, can isolated dysfunction of the internal anal sphincter lead to constipation? Only one definite condition involving this muscle has been proven to cause constipation: in a reported family an inherited myopathy of the internal anal sphincter caused proctalgia fugax and an inability to evacuate the rectum [42]. A strip myectomy of the sphincter relieved the symptoms.

## 1.5 Evacuation Proctography and Its Relationship to Defaecation

Defaecation involves a complex neural process which originates in the bowel or proximal to the rectum. By contrast, in evacuation proctography a contrast medium is placed into the rectum and the patient asked to evacuate. In the latter situation, rectal distension acts as part of the stimulus to emptying. In addition the subject increases intra-abdominal pressure, or "strains". This straining not only serves to increase intra-abdominal pressure but also may activate receptors in the bowel or rectum which initiate or facilitate rectal motor activity. Sphincter relaxation during proctography probably occurs by a conscious decision to evacuate, with a message via extrinsic pelvic nerves to the striated muscles to inhibit their activity and relax. Similar extrinsic neural control may cause internal anal sphincter relaxation.

## 1.6 Conclusion

The control of large bowel and sphincter function remains incompletely understood, and as a result the mechanism of most disorders of defaecation remains to be determined. An increased knowledge of these disorders will come from studying the relevant neural pathways, smooth muscle function and pelvic floor activity.

## References

1. Bueno L, Fioramenti J (1991) Cerebral and spinal control of gastrointestinal motor functions. In: Kamm MA, Lennard-Jones JE (eds) Gastrointestinal transit: pathophysiology and pharmacology. Wrightson Biomedical, Petersfield, pp 3–11
2. Smith JR, la Hann TR, Chesnut RM, Carino MA, Horita A (1977) Thyrotropin-releasing hormone: stimulation of colonic activity following intra-cerebroventricular administration. Science 196:660
3. Gue M, Jenien JL, Bueno L (1991) Conditional emotional response in rats enhances colonic motility through the central release of corticotrophin-releasing factor. Gastroenterology 100:964–970
4. Porreca F, Fiela A, Burks TF (1982) Spinal cord-mediated opiate effects on gastrointestinal transit in mice. Eur J Pharmacol 86:135–136

5. Porreca F, Mosberg HI, Hurst R, Hruby VJ, Burks TF (1984) Roles of mu, delta and kappa opioid receptors in spinal and supraspinal mediation of gastrointestinal transit effects and hot-plate analgesia in the mouse. J Pharmacol Exp Ther 230:341
6. Weber J, Denis P, Mihout B, Muller JM, Blanquart F, Galmiche JP, Simon P, Pasquis P (1985) Effect of brain-stem lesion on colonic and anorectal motility. Dig Dis Sci 30:419–425
7. Hinds JP, Eidelman BH, Wald A (1990) Prevalence of bowel dysfunction in multiple sclerosis. Gastroenterology 98:1538–1542
8. Klauser AG, Voderholzer WA, Heinrich CA, Schindlbeck NE, Muller-Lissner SA (1990) Behavioural modification of colonic function: can constipation be learned? Dig Dis Sci 35:1271–1275
9. Whitehead WE, Bosmajian L, Zanderman AB, Costa PT, Schuster MM (1988) Symptoms of psychological distress associated with irritable bowel syndrome. Gastroenterology 95:709–714
10. Drossman DA, McKee DC, Sandler RS, Mitchell CM, Cramer EM, Lawman BC, Bunger AL (1988) Psychological factors in the irritable bowel syndrome. Gastroenterology 95:701–708
11. Preston DM, Pfeffer J, Lennard-Jones JE (1984) Psychiatric assessment of patients with severe constipation. Gut 25:A582–583
12. Brook A (1991) Bowel distress and emotional conflict. J R Soc Med 84:39–42
13. Bleijenberg G, Kuypers HC (1987) Treatment of spastic pelvic floor syndrome with biofeedback. Dis Colon Rectum 30:108–111
14. Devroede G, Arhan P, Duguay C, Tetreault L, Akoury H, Perey B (1979) Traumatic constipation. Gastroenterology 77:1258–1267
15. Gunterberg B, Kewenter J, Petersen I, Stener B (1979) Anorectal function after major resections of the sacrum with bilateral or unilateral sacrifice of sacral nerves. Br J Surg 63:546–554
16. Narducci F, Bassotti G, Gaburri M, Morelli A (1987) Twenty-four hour manometric recording of colonic motor activity in healthy men. Gut 28:17–25
17. Cannon WB (1902) The movements of the intestines studied by means of the roentgen rays. Am J Physiol 6:251–277
18. Van der Sijp JRM, Kamm MA, Lennard-Jones JE (1991) Simulated defaecation: demonstration of colonic peristalsis with anal relaxation and rectal contraction. Gut 32:A563
19. Karaus M, Sarna SK (1987) Giant migrating contractions during defaecation in the dog colon. Gastroenterology 92:925–933
20. Kamm MA, Lennard-Jones JE, Thompson DG, Sobnack R, Garvie NW, Granowska M (1988) Dynamic scanning defines a colonic defect in severe idiopathic constipation. Gut 29:1085–1092
21. Schang JC, Devroede G (1988) Myoelectric propagating spike bursts in the sigmoid colon elicit the rectoanal inhibitory reflex. Gastroenterology 94:A403
22. Halls J (1965) Bowel content shift during normal defaecation. Proc R Soc Med 58:859–860
23. Bassotti G, Gaburri M, Imbimbo BP, Rossi L, Farrami F, Pelli MA, Morelli A (1988) Colonic mass involvements in idiopathic chronic constipation. Gut 29:1173–1179
24. Matsueda K, Yamato S, Kojima Y, Shoda R, Muraoka A, Kosaka H, Shimojo E, Umeda N, Oda T (1988) A new hypothesis on pathophysiology of diarrhoea and constipation types of irritable bowel syndrome. Gastroenterology 94:290
25. Milner P, Crowe R, Kamm MA, Lennard-Jones JE, Burnstock G (1990) Vasoactive intestinal polypeptide levels in the sigmoid colon are reduced in idiopathic constipation and increased in diverticular disease. Gastroenterology 99:666–675

26. Lincoln J, Crowe R, Kamm MA, Lennard-Jones JE, Burnstock G (1990) Levels of serotonin and 5-hydroxyindoleacetic acid are increased in the sigmoid colon in severe idiopathic constipation. Gastroenterology 98:1219–1225
27. Krishnamurthy S, Schuffler MD, Rohrman CA, Pope CE II (1985) Severe idiopathic constipation is associated with a distinctive abnormality of the colonic myenteric plexus. Gastroenterology 88:26–34
28. Rogers J, Misiewicz JJ, Henry MM (1987) Increased segmental activity and intraluminal pressures in the sigmoid colon of patients with the irritable bowel syndrome: a new manometric technique. Gut 28:A1344
29. Tucker DM, Sanstead HH, Logan GM, Klevay LM, Mahalko J, Johnson LK, Inman L, Inglett GE (1981) Dietary fibre and personality factors as determinants of stool output. Gastroenterology 81:879–883
30. Heaton KW (1991) Fibre and bulk preparations. In: Kamm MA, Lennard-Jones JE (eds) Gastrointestinal transit: pathophysiology and pharmacology. Wrightson Biomedical, Petersfield, pp 209–217
31. Sun WM, Read NW, Miner PB, Kerrigan DD, Donnelly TC (1990) The role of transient internal sphincter relaxation in faecal incontinence? Int J Colorectal Dis 5:31–36
32. Bartram CI, Turnbull GK, Lennard-Jones JE (1988) Evacuation proctography: an investigation of rectal expulsion in 20 subjects without defaecatory disturbances. Gastrointest Radiol 13:72–80
33. Shorvon PJ, McHugh F, Diamant NE, Somers S, Stevenson GW (1989) Defecography in normal volunteers: results and implications. Gut 30:1737–1749
34. Preston DM, Lennard-Jones JE (1985) Anismus in chronic constipation. Dig Dis Sci 30:413–418
35. Waldron D, Bowes KL, Kingma YJ, Cole DR (1988) Colonic and anorectal motility in young women with severe idiopathic constipation. Gastroenterology 95:1388–1394
36. Hallam RI, Williams NS, Melling J, Waldron DJ, Womack NR, Morrison JFB (1988) Treatment of anismus in intractable constipation with Botulinum A toxin. Lancet ii:714–716
37. Barnes PRH, Hawley PR, Preston DM, Lennard-Jones JE (1985) Experience of posterior division of the puborectalis muscle in the management of chronic constipation. Br J Surg 72:475–477
38. Kamm MA, Hawley PR, Lennard-Jones JE (1988) Lateral puborectalis division in the management of severe constipation. Br J Surg 75:661–663
39. Jones PN, Lubowski DZ, Henry MM, Swash M (1987) Is paradoxical contraction of puborectalis muscle of functional importance? Dis Colon Rectum 30:667–670
40. Duthie GS, Bartolo DCC, Miller R (1991) Laboratory tests grossly overestimate the incidence of anismus. Surgical Research Society (UK), abstract 42, Jan 1991
41. Kamm MA, Lennard-Jones JE (1990) Rectal mucosal electrosensory testing. Evidence for a sensory neuropathy in severe constipation. Dis Colon Rectum 33:419–423
42. Kamm MA, Hoyle CVH, Burleigh D, Law PJ, Swash M, Martin JE, Nicholls RJ, Northover JMA (1991) Hereditary internal anal sphincter myopathy causing proctalgia fugax and constipation. A newly identified condition. Gastroenterology 100:805–810

# 2 Ultrasound Anatomy of the Pelvic Floor

U. Hildebrandt

The development of rectal endosonography has had a dramatic impact on medical and surgical practice [1]. The technique has been demonstrated to be helpful in both benign and malignant conditions [2,3]. One of the so-called benign anorectal conditions is pelvic floor abnormalities [4]. These abnormalities are evaluated by a combination of barium enema studies, endoscopy, defaecography, anorectal manometry, electromyography of the external anal sphincter and the puborectalis muscle and colonic transit time assessment [5]. Because functional anorectal disorders are primarily evaluated by dynamic and functional investigations, it is not anticipated that endosonography will contribute significantly to their clarification. However, conditions like fistulas, abscesses and traumatic injuries of the sphincters, especially during childbirth, may extensively change the anatomy of the pelvic floor and cause functional disorders as a result. Surgery in the anorectal area has always relied on excellent anatomical delineation of the perineal structures, and there is hope that endosonographic technology will aid in the surgical management of the aforementioned conditions. There is no question that pathological alterations of the pelvic floor cannot be determined endosonographically unless the normal anatomy has been assessed by ultrasound. It is the purpose of this chapter to describe the anatomical details visible on ultrasound.

## 2.1 Equipment

Predominantly rigid probes have been available for rectal endosonography. They are inserted either blindly into the rectal lumen or through a rectoscope. The two types of scanner are linear and sector. Linear scanners have the disadvantage that the probe has to be rotated through 360° in the rectal lumen to completely evaluate adjacent organs and structures, and such scanners have not gained wide acceptance. Sector scanners are useful if the sector covers 360° but this is not usually the case. The superiority of 360° sector scanners lies in the fact that the rectum and its surroundings can be scanned continuously by simply drawing back the probe. The usual frequency of the transducer head is 7.5 MHz. It represents a compromise between resolution and penetration depth. With 7.5-MHz transducers the pelvis can be visualised completely up to the bony structures. There are probes with variable frequencies and others which combine linear and sector functions. Rigid probes should have the following features: (a) a shaft length of more than 20 cm for insertion of the probe through the rectoscope; (b) the option of using low and high frequencies for appropriate resolution of far and near targets; and (c) a radial scanner vertical to the longitudinal axis of the rectum. A 360° sector scanner is optimal. Just recently a flexible ultrasound colonoscope has become available. It has forward viewing optics and uses either a 7.5-MHz or a 12.0-MHz transducer with a motor-driven acoustic mirror providing a 320° sector scan.

## 2.2 Method of Examination

We use the rigid Brüel and Kjaer (Fig. 2.1) and the flexible Olympus (Fig. 2.2) instruments. In examinations with the rigid instrument the patient lies in the lithotomy position. Prior to the examination the rectum is evacuated with an enema. The lubricated probe is introduced into the rectum blindly. Following insertion of the probe, the rubber balloon which is attached over the transducer is filled with approximately 60 ml of degassed water to inflate the rectal wall.

During withdrawal of the probe the rectal, perirectal, anal and perianal regions are scanned in a continuous fashion. The water amount is reduced to about 5 ml when the transducer is placed within the anal canal. For examination of the anal canal a sonolucent plastic cap can be used instead of the balloon. Examinations with the flexible instrument are performed in the left lateral position. The examination technique is described in more detail elsewhere [6, 7].

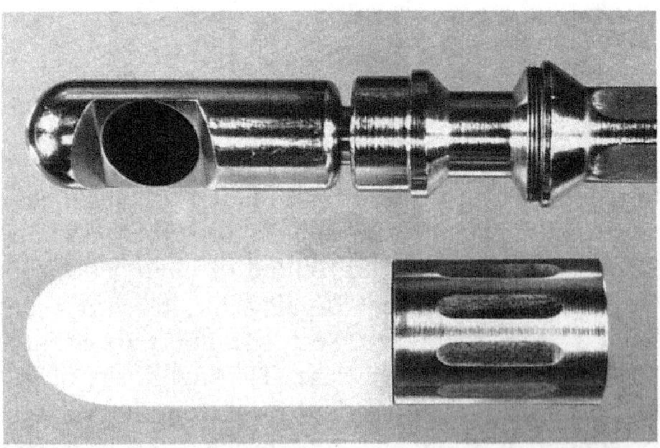

**Fig. 2.1.** Tip of the rigid Brüel and Kjaer probe, showing the 7.5-MHz transducer and, *below*, the sonolucent plastic cap which can be used instead of the balloon

## 2.3 Ultrasound Anatomy

### *2.3.1 The Perineum*

The perineum is the region overlying the inferior pelvic aperture. The posterior part, the anal triangle, contains the termination of the anal canal. The anterior part, the urogenital triangle, contains the external urogenital organs (Fig. 2.3). The boundaries of the perineum are the symphysis pubis, the inferior pubic rami, the ischial rami, the ischial tuberosities, the sacrotuberous ligaments and the coccyx.

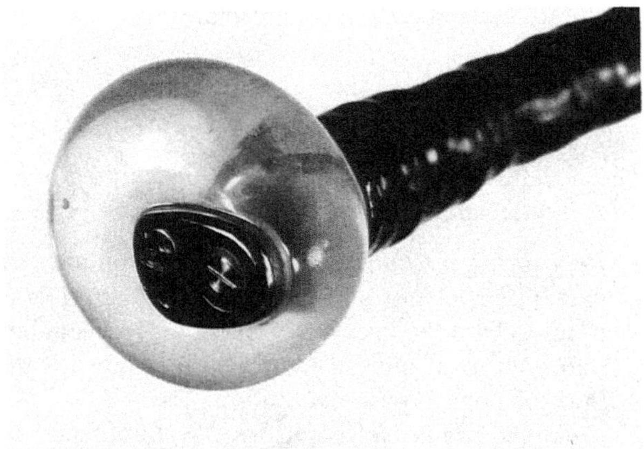

**Fig. 2.2.** Tip of the flexible Olympus ultrasound colonoscope with a water-filled balloon around the 7.5- or 12.0-MHz transducer. Forward viewing optics

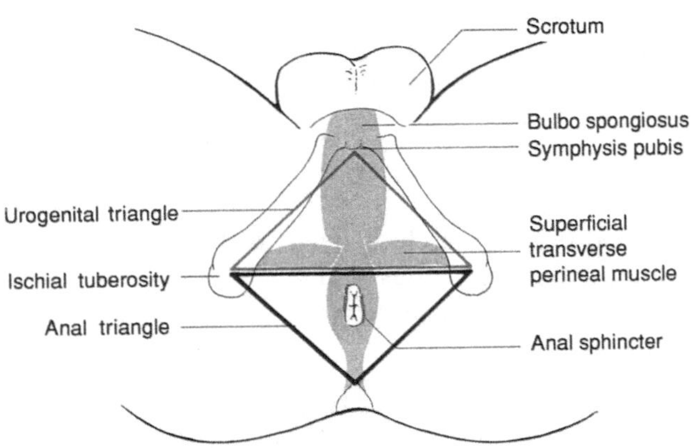


**Fig. 2.3.** Diagram illustrating the perineum (view in lithotomy position). A transverse line between the ischial tuberosities divides the perineum into the urogenital and the anal area

### *2.3.2 Muscles of the Pelvic Floor*

The two levator ani muscles and the two coccygeus muscles form the pelvic diaphragm. The levator ani muscles form most of the floor of the pelvic cavity, which separates it from the ischiorectal fossae. The levator ani muscles run postero-inferiorly from the anterolateral walls of the pubis minor and meet in the median plane from the posterior margin of the urogenital diaphragm to the coccyx. In the male the anterior fibres, passing inferior to the prostate and inserting into the central perineal tendon, constitute the levator prostatae muscle. In the female these fibres, crossing the sides of the vagina before ending in the central perineal tendon, constitute the pubovaginalis muscle.

#### *2.3.2.1 Levator Ani Muscles*

The levator ani muscles are divided into three parts: pubococcygeus, puborectalis and iliococcygeus.

1. *Pubococcygeus muscle* (Fig. 2.4). The pubococcygeus muscle is the main part of the levator ani. It arises from the pubis and runs posteromedially to insert into the coccyx and the anococcygeal ligament. In the female the pubococcygeus muscle encircles the urethra, vagina and anus and merges into the central perineal tendon.
2. *Puborectalis muscle* (Fig. 2.5). The puborectalis muscle is the part of the levator that lies medial to and at a more inferior level than the pubococcygeus muscle. Like the latter, it arises from the pubis and passes posteriorly. The muscles from the two sides loop around the posterior surface of the anorectal junction, forming a U-shaped rectal sling.
3. *Iliococcygeus muscle* (Fig. 2.6). The iliococcygeus muscle is the part of the levator ani that arises from the tendinous arch of the parietal pelvic fascia and the ischial spine. The muscle on each side passes medially and posteriorly and inserts into the coccyx and the anococcygeal ligament.

#### *2.3.2.2 Coccygeus Muscles*

Each coccygeus muscle lies against the posterior part of the iliococcygeus muscle and is continuous with it. The muscles form the posterior and smaller part of the pelvic diaphragm.

### ***2.3.3 Obturator Internus Muscle*** (Fig. 2.5)

The obturator internus muscle is a thick muscle that is situated partly within the pelvis minor. It covers most of the side wall of the pelvis minor and its origin is almost the entire internal surface of the anterolateral wall.

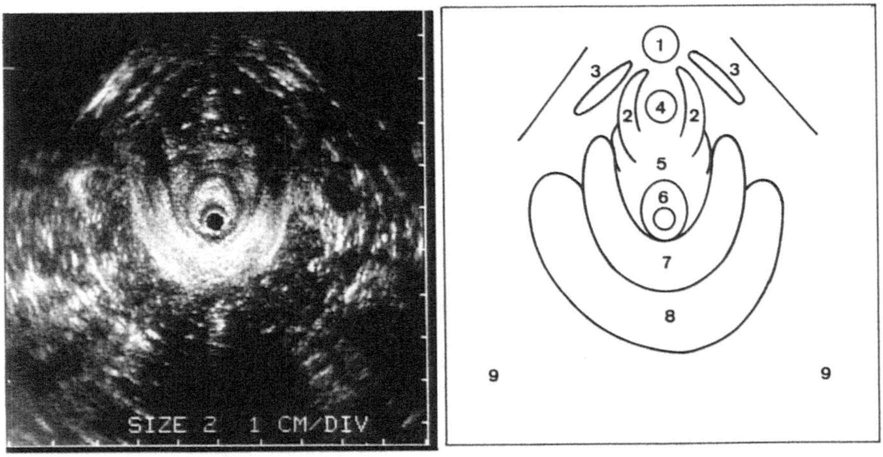


**Fig. 2.4.** Sonogram of the female perineum demonstrating the anal canal (*6*) and part of the levator ani muscle – the pubococcygeus muscle (*8*). Due to the funnel-shaped course of the levator ani, part of the ischiorectal fossa is visualized between the anal canal and the pubococcygeus muscle. Anteriorly to the vaginal orifice (*5*), the ischiocavernosus muscle (*3*) can be seen on both sides. It inserts into the crus of the clitoris (*1*). The bulbospongiosus muscle (*2*) arises from the central perineal tendon, passes around the vagina and inserts into the clitoris. *4*, urethra; *7*, ischiorectal fossa; *9*, gluteus maximus muscle

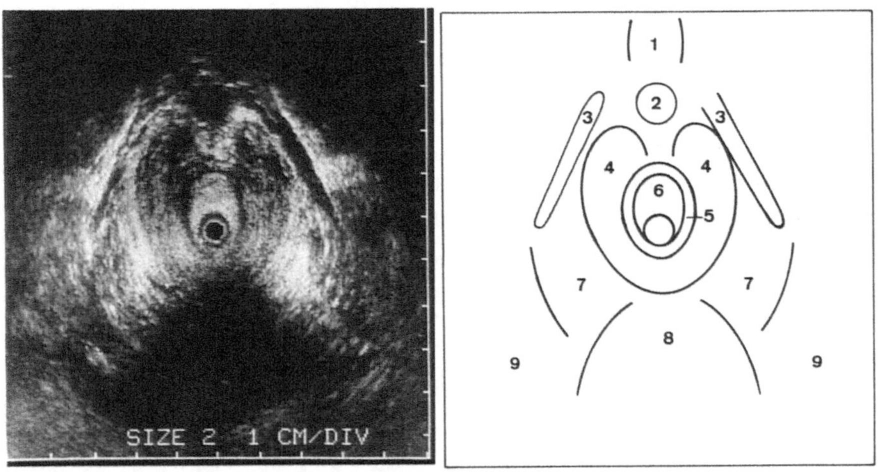


**Fig. 2.5.** Sonogram of the male perineum. Upper part of the anal canal with puborectalis muscle (*4*). The penis (*1*) and bulb of penis (*2*) are visualized anteriorly. The obturator internus muscle (*3*) is a thick muscle which is situated partly within the pelvis minor, where it covers most of the side walls. *5*, anorectal junction; *6*, mucosa; *7*, perianal fat; *8*, space between buttocks; *9*, gluteus maximus muscle

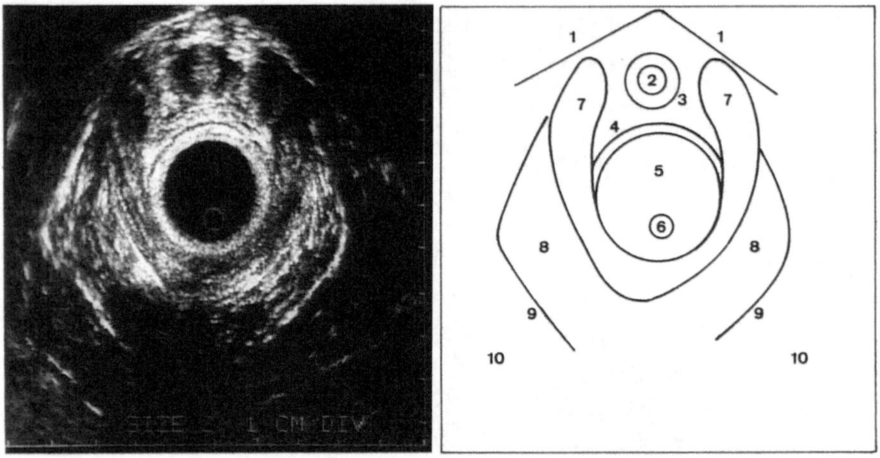


**Fig. 2.6.** Sonogram of the anorectal junction. The puborectalis muscle (*7*) is formed like a U-shaped sling. It lies at the point where the rectal ampulla narrows abruptly at the junction to the anal canal. For descriptive purposes three parts of the levator ani muscle are named: pubococcygeus, puborectalis (*7*) and iliococcygeus (*8*). The iliococcygeus muscle is the part of the levator ani that arises from the tendinous arch of the parietal pelvic fascia and the ischial spine. The muscle on each side passes medially and posteriorly and inserts into the coccyx and the anococcygeal ligament. *1*, symphysis; *2*, urethra; *3*, sphincter urethrae; *4*, rectal wall; *5*, rectal lumen; *6*, transducer; *9*, sacrotuberous ligament; *10*, gluteus maximus muscle

### *2.3.4 External Anal Sphincter* (Figs. 2.7, 2.8)

The external anal sphincter consists of three parts – subcutaneous, superficial and deep – but these parts are not distinctly separated from each other. The fibres of the external anal sphincter run from the central perineal tendon to the anococcygeal ligament.

### *2.3.5 Internal Anal Sphincter* (Figs. 2.7, 2.8)

The internal anal sphincter consists of a thickening of the circular smooth muscle of the intestine.

### *2.3.6 Ischiorectal Fossa* (Figs. 2.9, 2.10)

On each side of the anal canal and rectum there is a wedge-shaped space, the ischiorectal fossa. It is located between the skin of the anal region and the pelvic diaphragm. Because the levator ani is shaped like a funnel, the ischiorectal fossa on each side is wide inferiorly and narrow superiorly.

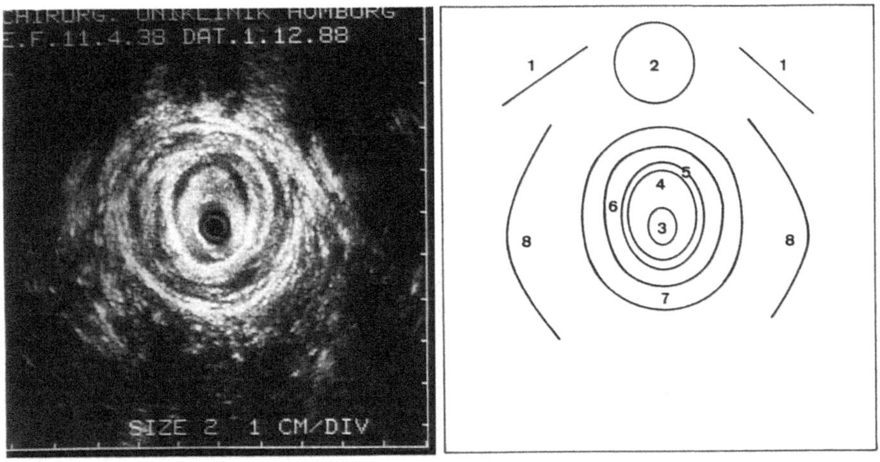


**Fig. 2.7.** Sonogram of the upper third of the anal canal. The internal anal sphincter (*5*) and the external anal sphincter (*7*) are surrounded by the levator ani muscles, which form the main part of the pelvic diaphragm. Because the levator ani is shaped like a funnel, it is covered in this section by the fat of the ischiorectal fossa (*8*). The bulb of the penis (*2*) is seen on the ventral side of the anal region. *1*, ramus pubis; *3*, anal canal with transducer; *4*, mucosa; *6*, fibrotic tissue

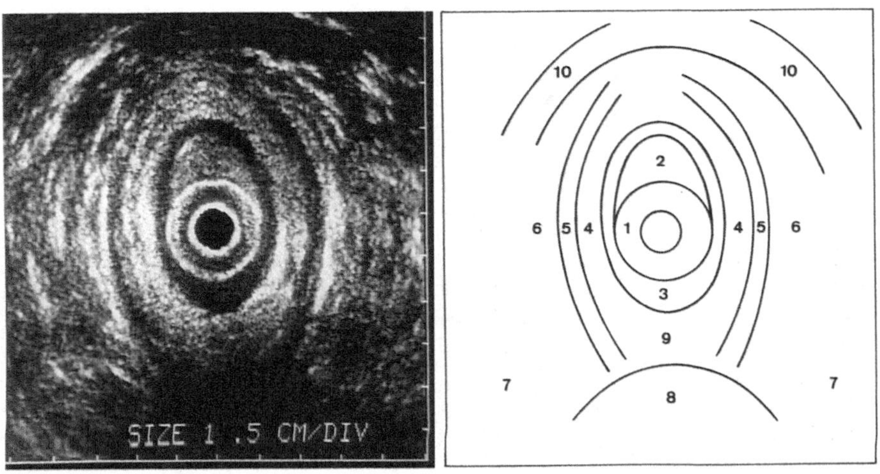


**Fig. 2.8.** Sonogram of the anal region. The transducer is positioned within the middle of the anal canal. The external anal sphincter (*5*) forms a broad band on each side of the anal canal which consists of three parts: subcutaneous, superficial and deep. These parts, however, are not distinctly separated from each other. The fibres of the external anal sphincter run from the central perineal tendon to the anococcygeal ligament (*9*). The internal anal sphincter (*3*) consists of a thickening of the circular smooth muscle surrounding the superior two-thirds of the anal canal. The transverse perineal muscle (*10*) inserts at the central perineal tendon. *1*, transducer; *2* mucosa; *4*, fibrotic tissue; *6*, ischiorectal fossa; *7*, gluteus maximus muscle; *8*, space between buttocks

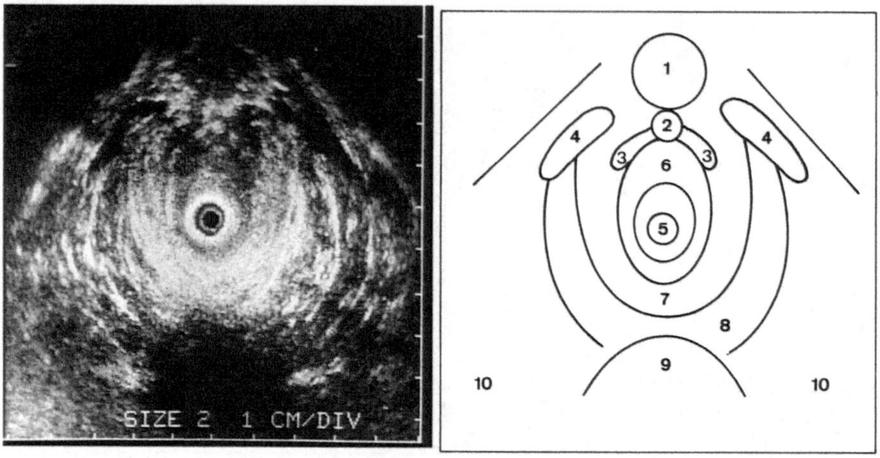


**Fig. 2.9.** Sonogram of the superficial perineal space in the male. There are three superficial perineal muscles: the superficial transversus perinei, the bulbospongiosus (*1*) and the ischiocavernosus (*4*). The last two are muscles of the penis. The transverse perineal muscle (*3*) and the levator ani (*7*) are anchored at the central perineal tendon (*2*). *5*, transducer; *6*, external anal sphincter; *8*, ischiorectal fossa; *9*, space between buttocks; *10*, gluteus maximus muscle

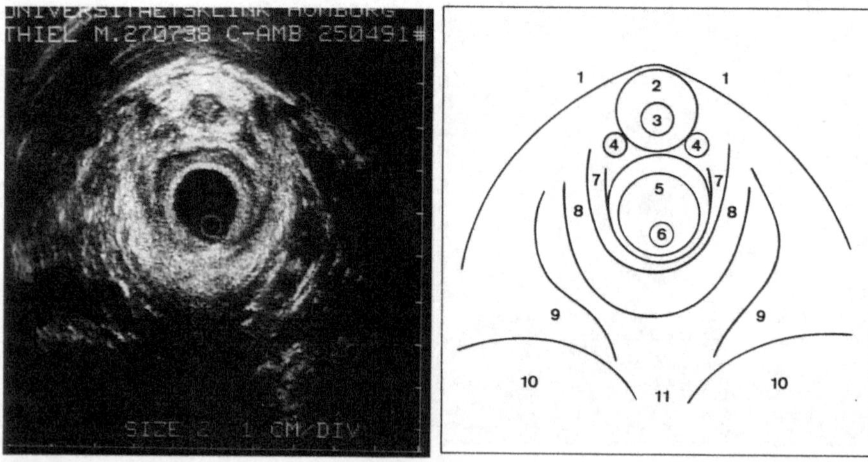


**Fig. 2.10.** Sonogram of the male perineum demonstrating a section through the roof of the penis. The urethra (*3*) is dilated within the bulb of the penis (*2*) (corpus spongiosum). The crus of the penis (*4*) consists of the corpus cavernosum. *1*, symphysis pubis; *5*, anal canal; *6*, transducer; *7*, *8*, external anal sphincter; *9*, ischiorectal fossa; *10*, gluteus maximus muscle; *11*, space between buttocks

### *2.3.7 Urogenital Diaphragm* (Figs. 2.6, 2.11–2.13)

The urogenital diaphragm is a thin sheet of striated muscle stretching between the two sides of the pubic arch. The urogenital diaphragm covers the anterior part of the inferior pelvic aperture. The most anterior muscle, the deep transversus perinei muscle, runs transversely, whereas the middle muscle, the sphincter urethrae muscle, encircles the urethra. Whereas in the male the sphincter urethrae muscle encircles the urethra, in the female it blends with the anterolateral walls of the vagina.

Anatomically the deep transversus perinei muscle consists of fibres posterior to the urethra. Endosonographically the muscle cannot be identified.

The central perineal tendon is a fibromuscular node located at the centre of the perineum. It is a landmark where the following muscles converge: transverse perineal muscles, bulbospongiosus muscle, fibres of the anal sphincter and levator ani muscles from both sides.

## 2.4 Clinical Applications of Ultrasound

Based on the normal endosonographic anatomy of the pelvic floor, anatomical alterations may be evaluated by ultrasound.

### *2.4.1 Surgical Trauma*

Surgical trauma may result in the development of incontinence. Incontinence related to surgery is usually the result of inappropriate division of the anorectal ring. Sphincter division through the puborectalis sling inevitably results in incontinence. Morphological alterations of the anal canal and the puborectalis muscle can be assessed by ultrasound.

### *2.4.2 Obstrectic Trauma*

Faecal incontinence may result from birth canal injury during vaginal delivery. This may result from median episiotomy (Fig. 2.14).

### *2.4.3 Accidental Trauma*

Trauma to the perineum can impair the sphincter mechanism. Impalement may result in division of the sphincter. Healing can entail excessive scar formation, resulting in an incompetent sphincter. Reconstructive sphincteric surgery for the different forms of trauma may be facilitated by the endosonographic assessment of the pelvic floor anatomy.

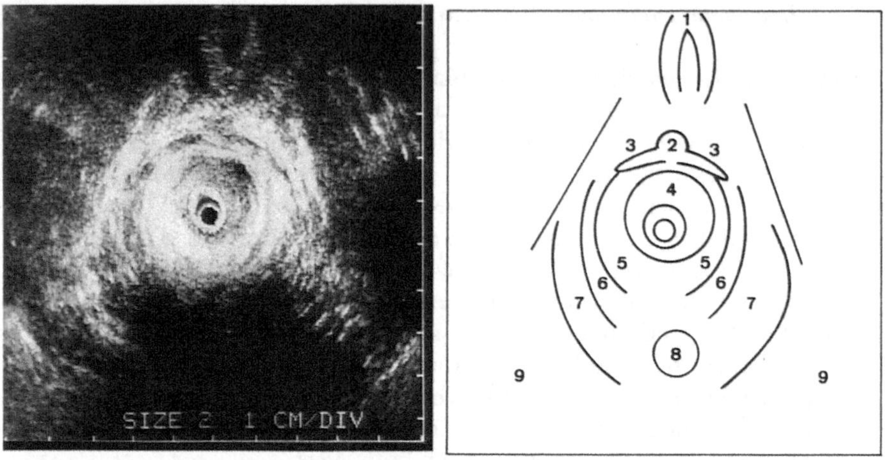


**Fig. 2.11.** Sonogram of the male perineal space demonstrating the bulbospongiosus muscle (*2*), which inserts together with the superficial perineal muscle and the external anal sphincter (*6*) at the central perineal tendon. *1*, penis; *3*, superficial perineal muscle; *4*, internal anal sphincter; *5*, fibrotic tissue; *7*, ischiorectal fossa; *8*, coccyx; *9*, gluteus maximus muscle

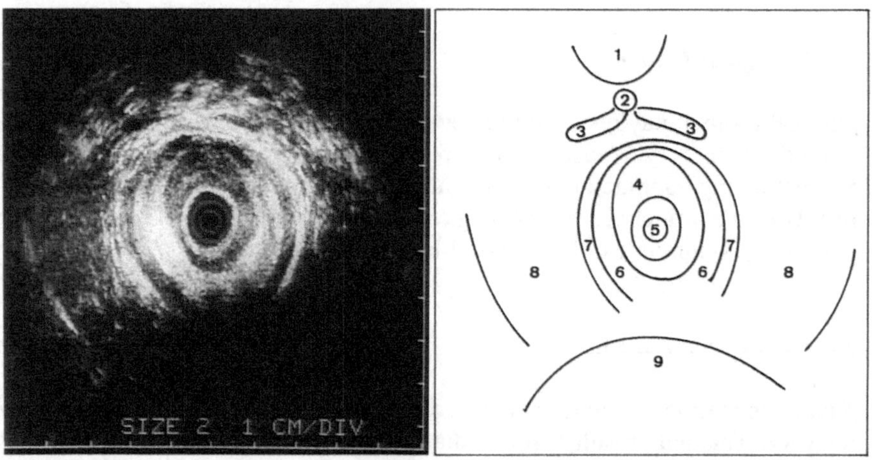


**Fig. 2.12.** Sonogram of the male perineal space. The central perineal tendon (*2*) is a fibromuscular node. The transverse perineal muscles (*3*) and fibres of the anal sphincter (*7*) and levator ani converge upon this point. *1*, bulb of penis; *4*, internal anal sphincter; *5*, transducer; *6*, fibrotic tissue; *8*, perianal fat; *9*, space between buttocks

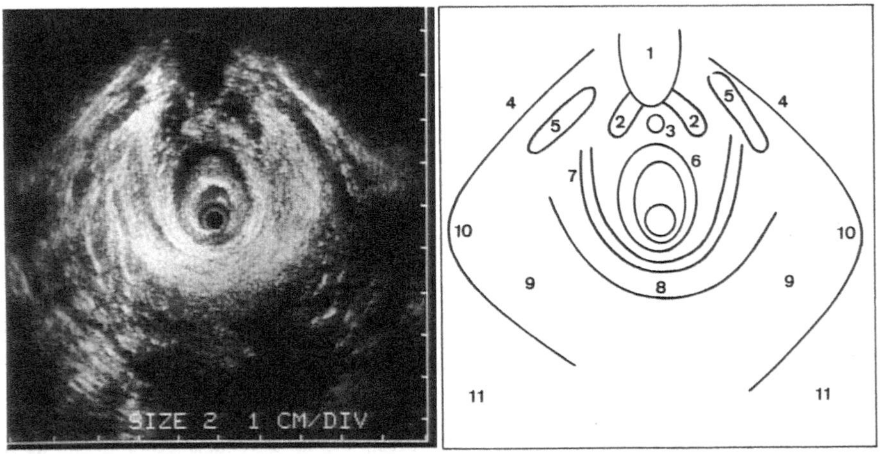


**Fig. 2.13.** Sonogram of the male perineum demonstrating one of the three superficial perineal muscles – the ischiocavernosus muscle (*5*). This muscle arises from the internal surface of the ischial tuberosity (*10*) and the ischial ramus (*4*) and passes anteriorly to the cavernous spaces (*2*) of the roof of the penis (*1*). *3*, corpus spongiosum; *6*, internal anal sphincter; *7*, external anal sphincter; *8*, ischiorectal fossa; *9*, levator ani; *11*, gluteus maximus muscle

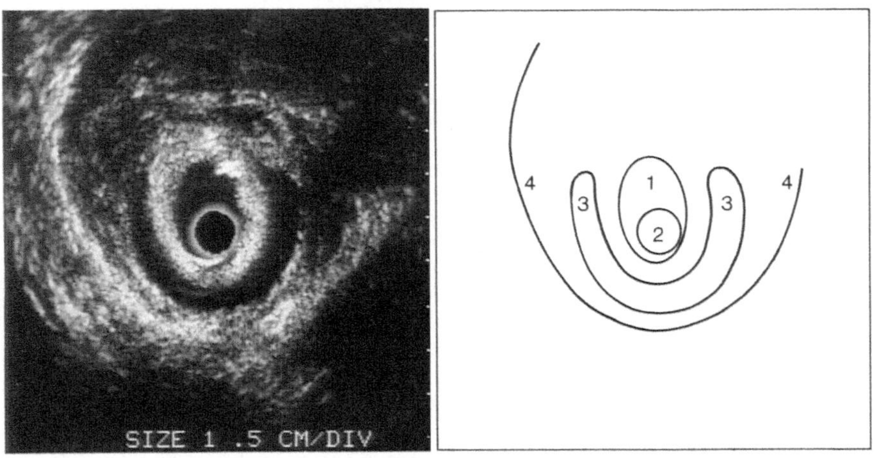


**Fig. 2.14.** Morphology of the external anal sphincter after obstetric trauma. The anterior part of the sphincter is divided by traumatic rupture. The internal anal sphincter appears U-shaped (*3*), indicating the defect anteriorly. *1*, anal canal; *2*, transducer; *4*, external sphincter

### *2.4.4 Differentiation of Abscesses*

Five types of anorectal abscess can be discerned by endosonography: perianal, ischiorectal, submucosal, intersphincteric and supralevator. It is important to distinguish the different types because their treatment differs. In particular, endosonography clarifies whether external or transrectal drainage would be appropriate.

### References

1. Hildebrandt U, Feifel G (1990) Endorectal sonography. Surg Annu 22:169–183
2. Hildebrandt U (1991) Local curative treatment of rectal cancer. Int J Colorectal Dis 6:74–76
3. Hildebrandt U, Feifel G, Ecker KW (1989) Rectal Endosonography. Baillieres Clin Gastroenterol 3:531–541
4. Kuijpers HC, Bleijenberg G (1985) The spastic pelvic floor syndrome: a cause of constipation. Dis Colon Rectum 28:669–672
5. Berman IR, Manning DH, Harris MS (1990) Streamlining the management of defecation disorders. Dis Colon Rectum 33:778–785
6. Feifel G, Hildebrandt U, Mortensen NJ (eds) (1990) Endosonography in gastroenterology, gynecology and urology. Springer, Berlin Heidelberg New York
7. Beynon J, Feifel G, Hildebrandt U, Mortensen NJ (1991) An atlas of rectal endosonography. Springer, Berlin Heidelberg New York

# 3 Pelvic Floor Stability and the Uterus

R. Hauck

## 3.1 Introduction

In the literature of defaecography, the pelvic floor is described as a muscular diaphragm. Functional control results from central innervation. Radiological imaging of this part of the pelvic floor can be performed indirectly by contrasting of the rectal wall, anal canal and crena anis according to the proposals of Mahieu and co-workers [1, 2] and others.

In this chapter consideration is given to the question of whether a description of functional changes of the muscular diaphragm alone during defaecation is sufficient to understand most of defaecation disorders or not. What is the influence of disturbances of the ligamental suspension of the uterus on defaecation disorders, and how can defaecography visualise the uterus and its suspension with regard to both static and functional anatomy?

## 3.2 Radiological Technique

In accordance with the method described in Sect 5.1, we favour complete contrast of the colon and, if possible, also of the terminal ileum. The position of the contrast-soaked vaginal tampon and other incorporated contrast (e.g. an intra-uterine contraceptive device, IUD) is of importance for interpretation.

## 3.3 Static Anatomy

The muscular pelvic floor consists mostly of the levator muscle. It is inserted into the pelvic bone and is funnel-shaped. It maintains its position if the rectum is filled or emptied. A kind of ceiling separates the rectum from other loops of colon or small intestine. This separating layer of tissue, the fascia pelvis superior, is the suspension of the uterus. It consists of a network of collagenous fibers and partly of smooth muscles. The fibers concentrate in the uterosacral, the uterolateral and the uterovesical ligaments.

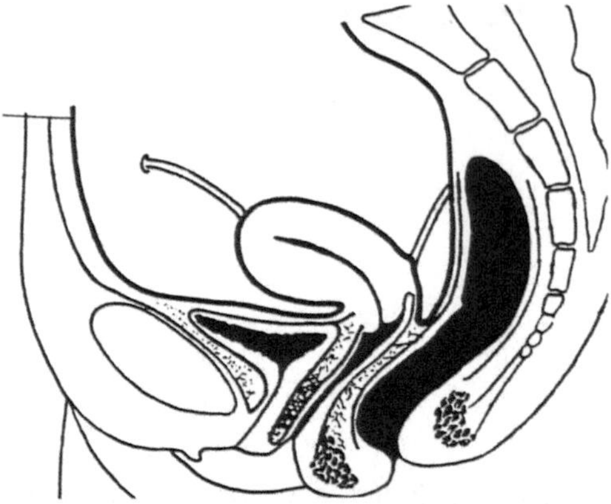

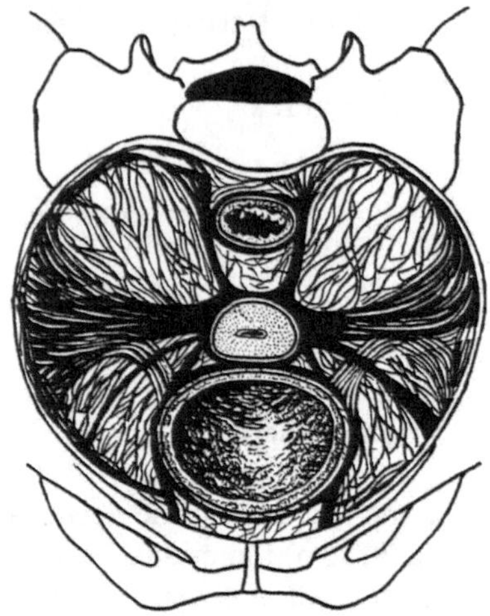

**Fig. 3.1** (*left*). Genital lamina – lateral view. (From Waldeyer [3])

**Fig. 3.2** (*right*). Genital lamina – frontal view. Note the "spider in a web" position of the uterus. (From Waldeyer [3])

In patients in the standing or sitting position, uterosacral ligaments have a more craniocaudal direction. Uterolateral ligaments have a more vertical position. Uterovesical ligaments are of lesser interest for defaecation disorders and have a more vertical position in continuation of the position of uterosacral ligaments. It is commonly accepted that this fascia pelvis superior forms an angle of about 45° with the pubococcygeal line.

Embedded in this network of collagenous fibers are nerves, following the uterosacral ligaments, and blood vessels, following the uterolateral ligaments. The Urethra is linked with uterovesical ligaments. Blood vessels and nerves pierce this fascia. The only structure which penetrates physiologically is the rectum. For our later functional considerations instead of fascia pelvis superior, we prefer to use the term "*Genitalplatte*" (genital lamina – author's translation) from Waldeyer [3] (Fig. 3.1).

The uterus is kept tightly in a central position, like a spider in the middle of a web (Fig. 3.2). Vertical movements of the uterus are possible. In 31 patients with IUDs investigated by us radiographically (unpublished work), the IUD, and thus the uterus, and the vaginal tampon placed nearest to the uterus moved in the same direction during defaecation.

In 400 patients without apparent pathological defaecographic alterations of general lamina, the range of IUD/vaginal tampon movement was 2.8 ± 1.1 cm. We consider this the possible movement of uterus and ligaments, bulging up when the rectum is filled and moving down during defaecation. When the rectum is empty, the genital lamina lie on the rectum like an inverted parachute.

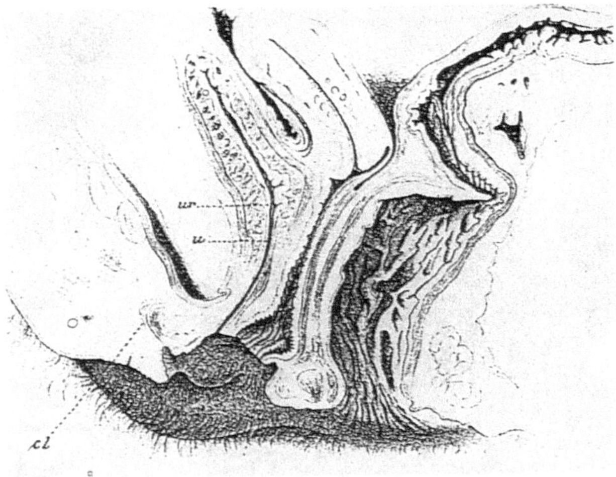


**Fig. 3.3.** Pouch of Douglas with its compartments: funnel-like cranial compartment, confined by rectum and uterus, and slot-like caudal compartment, confined by vagina and rectum. (From Richter [5])

As mentioned above, the only opening for the rectum is between the left and right uterosacral ligaments. Anatomically we find here the pouch of Douglas or excavatio recto uterina and recessus rectovaginalis (Fig. 3.3). From a defaecographic point of view, the pouch of Douglas is part of the occluding mechanism for the passage in genital lamina that should give way only for the rectum. In Sect. 3.4 (Functional Anatomy) we can demonstrate that this occluding mechanism functions in an anteflected as well as in a retroflected uterus. The pouch of Douglas consists of a slot-like part situated between the vagina and the rectum caudally. Cranially there may be a slot-like part between the retroflected uterus and rectum too, or a funnel-like part when the uterus is anteflected, as we will show later on [4].

## 3.4 Functional Anatomy

How does an increase in intestinal pressure during defaecation affect the ligamental pelvic floor described above?

"Strain of abdominal muscles provokes automatically a contraction of levator muscle and increase of pressure [on genital lamina]... and provokes furthermore a phenomenon which is called a lamellar effect... This effect is enforced by changing the vaginal situation around the deepest point of the levator plate... The strecking straightens the tight and inflexible collagenous fibers while elastic elements are activated to bring back collagenous framework into its former shape" [4].

Translated into a schematic drawing, straining pressure on genital lamina (Fig. 3.3a,b) in a case of retroflected uterus is shown as a thick arrow. When

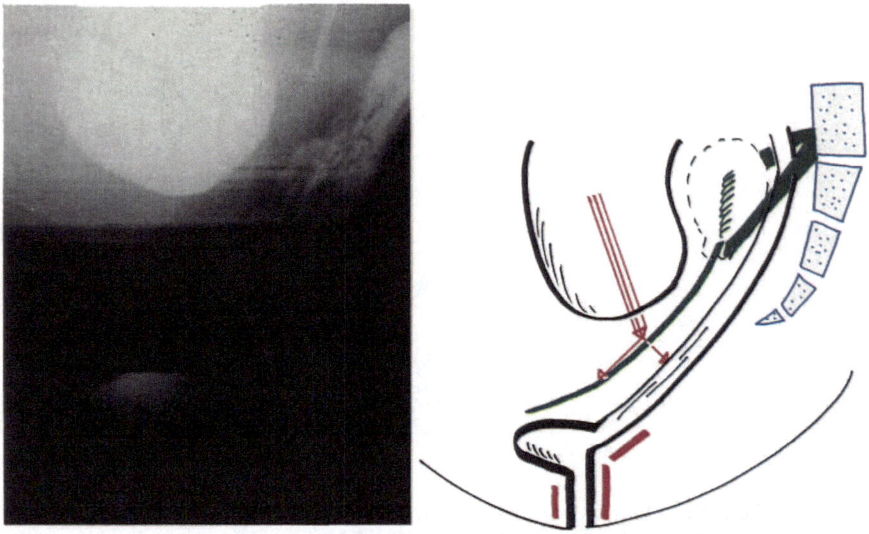

**Fig. 3.4.** Radiograph (*left*) and schematic drawing (*right*) of genital lamina clearly visible in a 48-year-old patient with retroflected uterus and IUD. The direction of intestinal pressure is marked by a *three-lined arrow*. The divided components of pressure (*single-lined arrows*) act towards the urinary bladder and the rectum[a]

it meets genital lamina, under a certain angle, it is divided into two components according to the parallelogram of forces.

One component has, therefore, an effect on the rectum and the muscular pelvic floor. When the rectum is filled, this component can help to evacuate this part of the colon. The other component is deflected towards the urinary bladder and pubis. The change in the vaginal situation is explained by this pressure component.

In our example (Fig. 3.4), the situation of the uterus is indicated clearly by the IUD, whereas a sigmoid loop follows intestinal pressure. In the corresponding radiograph the genital lamina can be recognized as a non-opacified tissure layer ventral to the rectum. A comparable situation can be shown in a patient without an IUD: we must assume that the retroflected uterus is in a relatively high position, that the sigmoid loop follows intestinal pressure, and a non-opacified tissue layer (Fig. 3.5) corresponds with the genital lamina. In the course of our considerations we should now regard the uterus situation as part of the occluding mechanism for the pouch of Douglas. It is clearly seen by consequent interpretation of lateral defaecographic exposures that the IUD-marked retro-flected uterus lies on the pouch of Douglas like a tap.

---

[a] The colours in the schematic drawings in this chapter and in chapters 16 and 17 indicate the following elements: *red lines*, musculature; *green*, ligamentum sacro-uterinum; *violet*, small intestine; *blue*, bones; *black*, contours of skin and large intestine, and vaginal tampon.

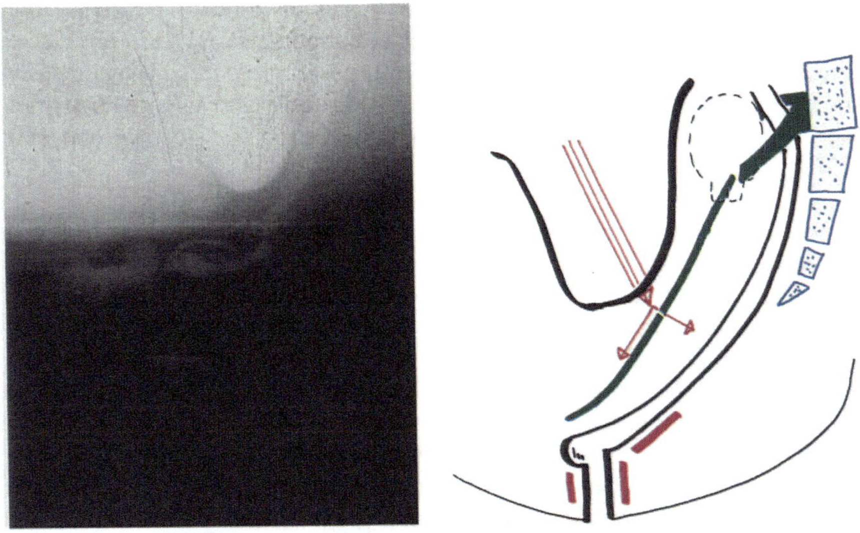

**Fig. 3.5.** Radiograph (*left*) and schematic drawing (*right*) of a 53-year-old patient with retroflected uterus. Same situation as in Fig. 3.4. The patient has no IUD. A rectocele is present

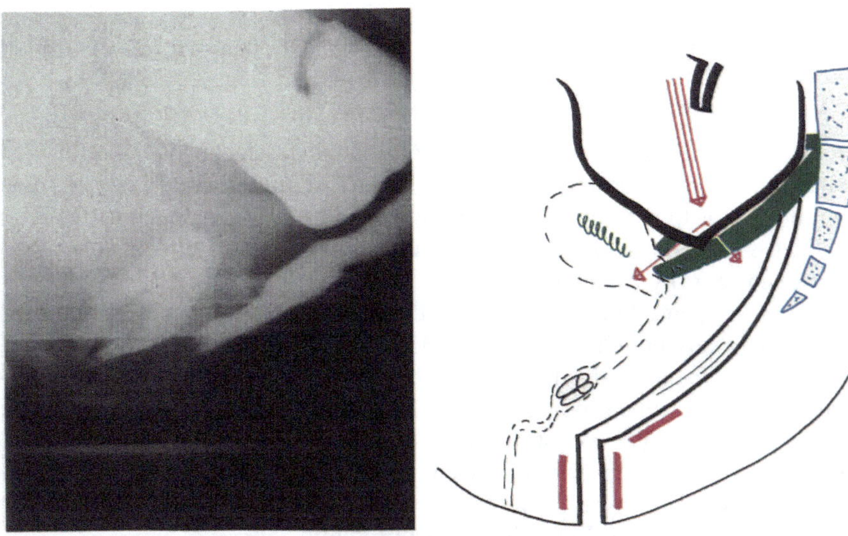

**Fig. 3.6.** Radiograph (*left*) and schematic drawing (*right*) of a 34-year-old woman with anteflected uterus and an IUD. A non-opacified layer indicates the location of the genital lamina. The *three-lined-arrows* indicate intestinal pressure. The divided components of pressure (*single-lined arrows*) act towards the urinary bladder and the rectum

Gynaecologists say that anteflected uterus is more frequent than retroflected. If we look at defaecograms in patients with IUD in anteflected uterus (Fig. 3.6) we see that under intestinal pressure, the funnel-like superior part of the pouch of Douglas is wide open and filled with sigmoid loop. The occluding mechanism is done by pressing the slot-like part (Fig. 3.3) down and against the rectum.

*Functional Anatomy in Patients with an Open Pouch of Douglas.* Since we have not found any paper studying Douglas pouch mechanism in defaecograms, we deduct from gynaecological literature [4] that an open pouch of Douglas is a requirement for the formation of an enterocele. Only then does intestinal pressure act directly on the rectum without being divided into separate components (Figs. 3.7, 3,8). In defaecograms, the formation of enterocele varies as described in Chap. 17. We found six enteroceles in patients with defaecographic disorders and with IUD. In Fig. 3.8 (left), a schematic drawing shows undivided intestinal pressure (arrow). The distance between uterus and rectum is great and air bubbles prove small intestine as content of the hernial sac.
Our IUD patients with enteroceles are so few that the criteria used by us for the probable diagnosis "aperture of the pouch of Douglas" are subject to possible alterations of:

- Vertical position of the uterus
- Sigmoid loop overlaying rectum in normal position before bowel evacuation
- Very flat kyphotic curve of os coccygis

In all cases we described, the ligaments of the fascia pelvis superior were untouched. Pelvic floor stability was regarded under conditions of functioning or not functioning of occluding mechanism of the pouch of Douglas. An extreme case is given when the uterus is removed and ligaments are destroyed, e.g. by tumor surgery (Fig. 3.9).
There is no genital lamina because of the destruction of ligaments, and there is no longer any pouch of Douglas: the uterus is removed, the vaginal stump is no longer fixed by ligaments, and the stump is moved away by intestinal pressure. A peritoneal pouch is smoothed and unfolded in this way.
In this case, no deflection of intestinal pressure is possible. Consequently the pressure affects the muscular pelvic floor and anal canal directly. A vaginal tampon pushed far away, a retocele, and even a forward deflection of anal canal, as illustrated in Fig. 3.9, are symptomatic.

## 3.5 Conclusion

The fascia pelvis superior is functionally shown as a deflecting membrane for intestinal pressure. It protects the muscular pelvic floor from the direct and

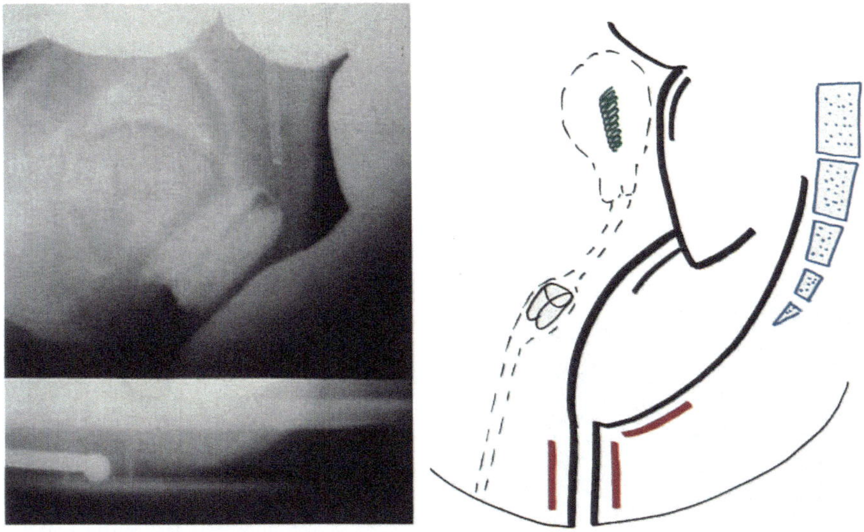

**Fig. 3.7.** Radiograph (*left*) and schematic drawing (*right*) of a 29-year-old female. Defaecography in the lateral projection and with the patient at rest shows no abnormal aspect. The anatomical locations of a contrast-soaked tampon and an IUD are visible

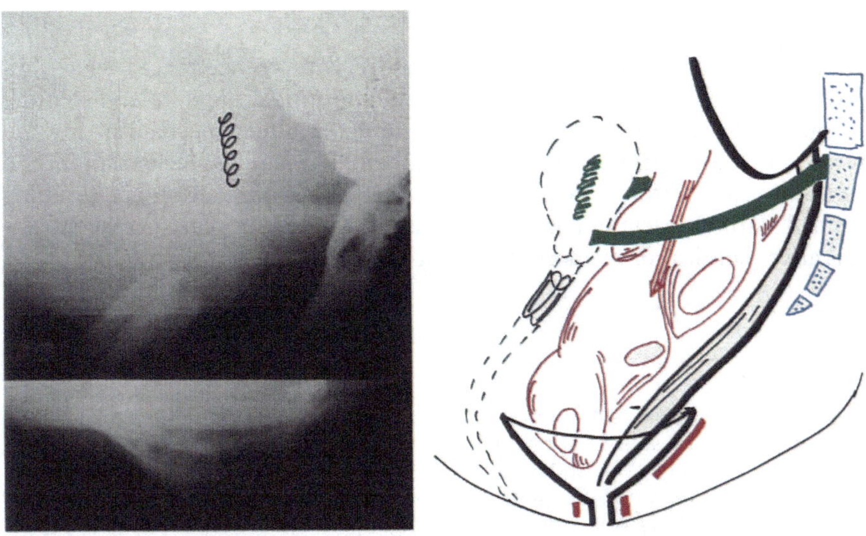

**Fig. 3.8.** Radiograph (*left*) and schematic drawing (*right*) of the same patient as in Fig. 3.7. The *three-lined arrow* indicates intestinal pressure. The long or distended uterosacral ligaments make possible the opening of the pouch of Douglas and the entry of small intestine into it

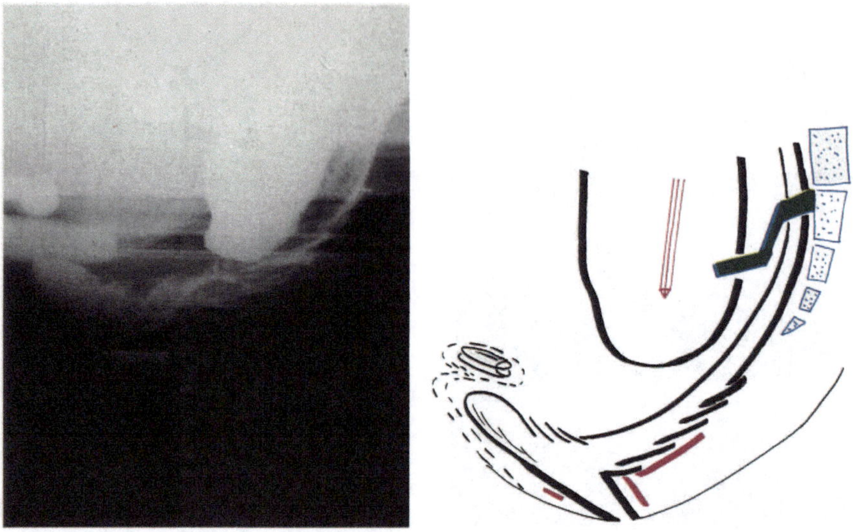

**Fig. 3.9.** Radiograph (*left*) and schematic drawing (*right*) of a 58-year-old patient with destroyed and resected ligaments because of tumorous infiltration. Intestinal pressure (*three-lined arrow*) acts to bend the anal canal forward and to press a rectocele in the direction of the vagina. A vaginal tampon is pushed away. No deflection of intestinal pressure is possible

pathological influence of intestinal pressure with consequences which are given in more detail in Chap. 17. Deflecting intestinal pressure and splitting up its unidirectional force is an important occluding mechanism for the pouch of Douglas (preventing enterocele) and evacuating mechanism for the rectum. With better understanding of the defaecation disorders resulting from disturbed fascia pelvis superior, it is more likely that successful conservative, surgical or gynaecological forms of treatment will be found.

## References


1. Mahieu P, Pringot J, Bodart P (1984) Defecography: I. Description of a new procedure and results in normal patients. Gastrointest Radiol 9:247–251
2. Mahieu P, Pringot J, Bodart P (1984) Defecography: I. Contribution to the diagnosis of defecation disorders. Gastrointest Radiol 9:253–261
3. Waldeyer A (1967) Anatomie des Menschen, part I. De Gruyter, Berlin
4. Richard W, TE Linde (1962) Opertative gynecology. John Hopkins University Press, Baltimore
5. Richter K (1985) In: Käser O, Friedberg V, Ober KG, Thomsen K, Zander J (eds) Gynäkologie und Geburtshilfe, Bd III, Teil 1, 4.1–4.35

# 4 Case History and Clinical Examination

P. Buchmann

Despite the many sophisticated methods for investigation of the anoerctum described in this book, the case history and clinical examination are of the greatest importance and together constitute a compulsory first procedure. They are of crucial interest not only for the clinician but also for the radiologist investigating functional disorders because many alterations are only demonstrable when especially searched for.

## 4.1 Case History

Questioning of patients attending a rectal clinic is divided into two parts; the first concerns less recent case history and the second, the development of symptoms and actual complaints. The first part includes questions regarding:

Mental disorders
General neurological disorders
Spinal injury
Inflammatory bowel disease
Drugs
Surgery (local, bowel)
Obstetric and gynaecological history

The obstetric and gynaecological history (number of children, how they were delivered, hysterectomy: vaginal or transabdominal) is of particularly great importance. In addition, questioning in respect of urinary disorders provides information on the anterior part of the pelvic floor and, in males, the condition of the prostate.
The second part of the questioning requires guidance of patients because many of them are embarrassed to talk about their proctological problems and only mention the one symptom from which they suffer most. In order to overcome taboos it is best to follow a questionnaire that covers all possible symptoms and disorders (Table 4.1; Appendix). With the knowledge so obtained, it is often possible to reach a definite diagnosis.
The location, frequency, duration and triggering of pain are all indicative of its cause. Sharp pain during and shortly after defaecation is associated with a

**Table 4.1.** Most important points in a proctological case history

| |
|---|
| Pain |
| Bleeding |
| Discharge |
| Pruritus ani |
| Swelling and tumor |
| Prolapse |
| Defaecation |
| - Bowel habits |
| - Incontinence |

lesion in the anal canal (e.g. anal fissure or, rarely, an intersphincteric abscess). If the pain is more constant, external and associated with a circumscribed swelling, a thrombosis in the external haemorrhoidal venous plexus is most probable. Slowly increasing perianal pain is caused by an abscess or the retention of pus in a pre-existing fistula tract.

A constant but dull pain in the anorectum is related to an inflammation in the anus or rectum (cryptitis, proctitis) or, if it occurs mainly during defaecation, to internal haemorrhoids. A carcinoma reaching deep layers of the bowel wall or sphincter ani must not be overlooked, and some men with prostatitis erroneously contact a proctologist. Cramp-like pains are fortunately rate but difficult to treat because conditions such as anismus or proctalgia fugax may have fine-sounding names but are still poorly defined.

As regards bleeding, the amount ranges from smears on the toilet paper in patients with erosions and perianal dermatitis or a fissure, through drops of blood or blood stains on stools in patients with haemorrhoids or rectal carcinoma, to bloody diarrhoea during acute proctitis or colitis and finally bleeding in sufficient quantities to cause anemia in the presence of diverticular disease or haemangioma.

The colour of the blood and the degree of mixture with stool depend on the distance from the origin of the bleeding to the anus and the severity of the bleeding. Bright red blood in small amounts originates from the anus and rectosigmoid. The higher its source, the more the blood is mixed with stool and the darker is its colour; it may even be black when the source is a gastroduodenal ulcer. Only shock-producing bleeding results in a bright red clotted blood loss even when the origin is high.

In my experience, soiled pants and anal symptoms are usually the result of anal discharge rather than poor hygiene. The loss of some mucus and faeces is caused by incomplete closure of the anus (e.g. in proctitis or after anal surgery, especially fistulotomy) and results in perianal dermatitis with erosions and itching. Some patients with an anal fistula suffer from the same symptoms.

Beside general conditions (e.g. psychogenic or allergic disease), pruritus ani may be due to a local skin alteration (e.g. perianal dermatitis including

eczema and mycosis, or psoriasis). However, sometimes the aspect is quite normal. It is very difficult to help these patients. Many of them are impassioned anal cleaners or use a high-pressure water cleaning device to fill the rectal ampulla with water, which gradually escapes.
A diffuse painful perianal swelling originates from an abscess. An acutely appearing painful tumor at the anal verge is caused by a thrombosis in the external rectal venous plexus. The rare incarcerated haemorrhoidal prolapse with thrombosis of the internal plexus is easily differentiated from the latter lesion because of the visible mucosa. However, most tumors are painless and slow growing. They become a source of discomfort upon infiltrating sphincter muscles (malignoma) or interfering with closure of the anal canal (e.g. malignoma, condylomata acuminata, hypertrophic papilla). The most common of all alterations are "skin tags," harmless skin folds of different size that appear with age or during the development of an anal fissure. In Crohn's disease a typical lymphoedematous swelling occurs, indicating active inflammation in the anus or intestinally.
A prolapse is classified according to the modified Miles grading system:

Grade 1: endoscopically visible
Grade 2: visible, with spontaneous repositioning
Grade 3: visible, digital repositioning needed
Grade 4: visible, repositioning impossible

Patients suffering from grade 3 or 4 prolapse (haemorrhoidal, anal or rectal) know well what their doctor is talking about, but patients without prolapse or with only low-grade prolapse normally do not understand the question concerning prolapse. The same is true for incontinence.
In proctology defaecation habits are of central importance. One should enquire regarding:

1. Frequency ("How often do you visit the toilet?")
2. Consistency
   - hard
   - soft (which is normal)
   - semisolid
   - watery
   - variable
3. Urgency of defaecation (with or without incontinence)
4. Feeling of incomplete evacuation
5. Straining needed
   - with constipation
   - with soft stool
6. Special manoeuvre needed (e.g. use of finger)
7. Intake of drugs: see Table 4.2

A record of bowel habits may be helpful but should be maintained only for a limited time because of the risk of psychological fixation on bowel

**Table 4.2.** Drugs influencing bowel habits. (Nicholls and Glass [4])

| Diarrhoea | Constipation | Bleeding |
|---|---|---|
| Aperients | Opiates | Anticoagulants |
| Antibiotics | Anticholinergics | Drugs causing marrow depression; cytotoxics: immunosuppressants |
| Magnesium antacids | Ganglion blockers | |
| Digitalis | Antidepressants (MAO inhibitors; some tricyclics) | |
| | Iron | |
| | Calcium, aluminium antacids | |

problems. overlooking minor disorders is often more beneficial than close observation.

Constipation is so common in Western civilisation that one might think it a normal condition. However, many diseases are related to hard and infrequent stool. The most important measure to overcome constipation is a high-fibre diet with sufficient fluid [i.e. at least 3 dl of fluid per soupsoon (10 g) of bran]. In therapy-resistant cases, more detailed exploration is needed (see Chaps. 13 and 18).

Urgency of defaecation forces the patient always to stay close to a toilet. In some the urge is so strong that incontinence occurs before the lavatory is reached. Many otherwise continent persons experience incontinence with urgency during an attack of acute enteritis. In inflammatory bowel disease, too, this symptom disappears with control of the episode. When the cause of urgency is unknown, i.e. it is not simply a question of acute diarrhoea, a colonoscopy should first be performed (see Chap. 11).

The feeling of incomplete evacuation is typical for a rectocele. During straining the rectocele is filled and at the end of defaecation it is emptied into the upper anal canal, eliciting a new urge. Use of a finger to push the posterior vaginal wall backward during emptying demonstrates the causality of the rectocele (i.e. weakness of the rectovaginal septum). However, the same feeling occurs in other conditions when the upper anal canal is widened after defaecation (e.g. hypertrophic papillae, haemorrhoids, rectal adenoma). Patients should be discouraged from practising manoeuvres with the finger because of the damage they cause to the anal lining (as can be observed in paraplegics) and the development of a psychological obsession to continue doing so. Excessive straining in the absence of hard stool is caused by an outlet obstruction. There are several possible reasons for such an obstruction: enterocele (see Chaps. 15 and 17), anal dysplasia (see Chap. 20), tumor or anal spasm (e.g. with an anal fissure).

Incontinence ranges from the discharge of mucus to uncontrolled evacuation of solid stool. It is of interest to learn how it came about (e.g. after surgery, slowly increasing, after delivery) and whether it entails flatus or watery, semisolid or solid stool. Further questions include:

1. Is the urge to defaecate so great that retention is impossible?
2. Is a prolapse part of the disorder?
3. Is there any relationship to food intake?

With regard to further exploration and treatment, see Chaps. 14 and 19.

## 4.2 Inspection

The position of the patient for examination depends on the doctor's routine. I favor the left lateral position with the knees drawn up because the patient then does not feel exposed. However, for some conditions the lithotomy position may be preferable. Some proctologists use the knee-elbow position (with a special examination table), which is most convenient for the doctor but also most inconvenient for the patient.

Inspection starts with checking the pants, perianal skin, and, if used, the sanitary towel for soiling with stool, pus or blood. The patient is asked when he washed last. Before cleaning the perianal region we observe whether it is dry or wet. Colour and superficial skin lesions (e.g. erosions, leucokeratosis) are recognised. We then look for tumors (e.g. skin tags, condylomata acuminata, cancer), deformity of the anus by scarring, and fistula openings. Very rarely we detect a crab louse or vermicule (oxyuriasis).

Especially in children but also in adults the positioning of the anus may be abnormal; in particular the anus may be anteriorly displaced (see Chap. 20) and eccentrically positioned in the perianal pigmentation. Lack of fixation of the upper anal canal to the coccyx results in the anus being pulled forward by the puborectalis sling and the subcutaneous part of the external sphincter forming a wall between the anal opening and the posterior commissure of the vaginal introitus or, in men, the scrotum. As a final step in the inspection we ask the patient to "squeeze" in order to ascertain whether the correct muscles (not the gluteus) are used, and also to "push down" in order to observe whether a prolapse is produced.

## 4.3 Perianal Palpation

The anal surrounding is carefully palpated in a search for painful areas (abscess) or tumours (thrombosis) and a subcutaneous fistula tract. Usually in perianal abscesses fluctuation is missed until the cavity reaches an enormous size. Painless skin indurations and hard skin tags are suspicious for a carcinoma and need to be biopsied; cartilaginoid skin tags are typical for Crohn's disease and are better left alone.

With a cotton carrier the sensitivity of the skin is compared with other parts of the body. The border of an area of impaired innervation can be easily determined by moving the cotton plug slowly and serpentinely away from the anus in different directions. With the wooden end of the cotton carrier the cutaneo anal reflex can be elicited. Scratching the perianal skin elicits a sphincter contraction.

## 4.4 Rectal Digital Exploration

Upon introducing the well-lubricated index finger into the anal canal, the groove between the internal and external sphincter muscle is palpable just proximal to the anocutaneous line. A sharp pain at this point, especially posteriorly or anteriorly, usually originates from an anal fissure; much more rarely an intersphincteric abscess is responsible. The pain-induced spasm often prevents further examination, but use of a local anaesthetic ointment solves this problem.

In the middle of the anal canal, pathology on the dentate line (e.g. inner opening of a fistula, hypertrophic papillae) is palpable. In anal dysplasia a posterior gap caused by the absence of the middle sphincter muscle loop can be felt.

The finger reaches the rectal ampulla; a search is then conducted for polyps, carcinoma, a solitary rectal ulcer, or a supralevator or Douglas abscess, and the prostate or portio is checked. It has to be kept in mind that internal haemorrhoids are not palpable! The posterior part of the pelvic floor (levator ani muscle) is palpated to identify any muscle gaps. The patient is then asked to push down, which may provoke a rectal intussusception or enterocele. With the tip of the index finger positioned posteriorly at the internal end of the anal canal, the patient is asked to retain as strongly as possible so that correct innervation and strength of the puborectalis sling can be ascertained.

The approximate length of the anal canal to the tip of the coccyx is established by palpation: it is decreased in descending perineum syndrome (Fig. 4.1) and increased in anal dysplasia (see Chap. 20). The firmness of the

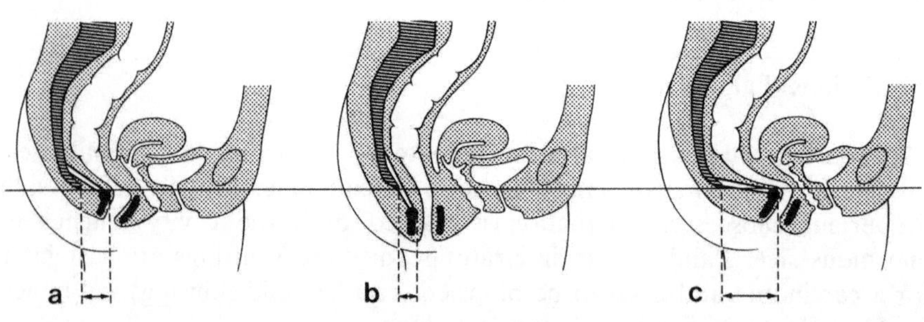


**Fig. 4.1a–c.** The pelvic floor. **a** Normal position of the puborectalis sling and normal distance between it and the coccyx. **b** Caudal positioning of the anus and decreased distance from the puborectalis sling to the coccyx. **c** Anal dysplasia with an increased distance from the puborectalis sling to the coccyx and perineal wall formation between the anus and vagina

anterior rectal wall and posterior vagina is controlled by pushing the phalangette ventrally. In the presence of a rectocele the posterior vaginal wall appears in the vaginal introitus. Turning the finger 180° and again placing the tip on the puborectalis sling (the inner end of the anal canal), the resting and squeeze pressure can be estimated. When the stretched finger is moved around in the anus, a healthy sphincter always lies close to the glove. Persistence of an open anal canal after the finger is withdrawn indicates spinal damage between T12 and L3.
Finally the length of the anal canal is measured (normal length: 3–4 cm) while withdrawing the finger, and the exploration is completed by checking the colour of stool and looking for possible blood smears on the glove.

## 4.5 Proctoscopy and Sigmoidoscopy

Although theoretically the rectum should be empty most of the time, sigmoidoscopy is rarely possible without an enema. Therefore some proctologists ask the patient to introduce a microenema before he enters the examination room. This carries a small risk of effacing minor alterations (e.g. anal soiling, blood smears) and of producing slight oedema of the mucosa but eases the exploration.
The aim of endoscopy is to visualise the palpated and suspected findings with the possibility of biopsy, collection of faeces etc. or therapy (e.g. coagulation, rubber-band ligation). If the case history and clinical examination have been complete up to this point, accidental findings are rare.
The best instrument for investigating the anal canal and lowermost part of the rectal ampulla is a short proctoscope (anoscope) (see Chap. 11). The rest of the rectum and the distal sigmoid colon can be examined by a rigid sigmoidoscope (rectoscope) or flexible endoscope (see Chap. 11). The advantages of the rigid instrument in terms of time saving and cost are to some extent offset by the disadvantage that due to pain the tube often cannot be inserted farther than 15 cm, i.e. just up to the rectosigmoid junction.
Utilising one's knowledge of the anatomy of the anal canal, the endoscope is introduced pointing to the umbilicus, followed by a sharp bend toward the lower sacrum to enter the rectal ampulla. After full introduction the instrument is slowly retracted, insufflating air if possible. In proctoscopy the retraction is interrupted at the level of the internal rectal venous plexus and the scope is moved slightly up and down to produce a prolapse of the piles into the instrument. If the patient is asked to push during extraction of the scope, retention of a procidentia by the sphincter contraction is impossible.
Thus even an extremely embarrassed patient pushing and squeezing at the same time is outwitted and demonstrates a haemorrhoidal prolapse or rectal intussusception.

With endoscopy of the distal part of the gastrointestinal tract the routine clinical examination ends. In most patients these investigations are sufficient; when they are not, a great variety of methods exist for more detailed investigation. The following chapters deal with these techniques.

## 4.6 Specimen Sampling

Either biopsy is performed during endoscopy using a forceps or an open biopsy is performed. Distal to the dentate line, local anaesthesia is mandatory. Normally the specimen is transported in a formalin-filled sample bottle. Only a rather large biopsy specimen is suitable for frozen section.

In the distinction between benign and malignant lesions, cytology is sometimes helpful. Inguinal lymph nodes and subcutaneous and low pararectal tumours are best suited for cytological analysis. A specially designed syringe is employed in the technique. Following insertion of the needle and aspiration, the aspirate is expressed onto a slide, smeared and plunged into a fixation solution prior to transport.

Skin specimens to identify fungal infection are best taken with a knife, scraping several times over the lesion and putting the scrapings without any stabilizer into a sterile test tube. Avoid contact with lubricant gel because evaluation might be distorted. In fact, however, this examination is usually unnecessary since (a) as a rule, any skin lesion immediately becomes infected by a fungus, and (b) successful treatment of perianal dermatitis normally cures the fungal infection too.

Culturing pus from an abscess or fistula again is of limited value. If bacteriology demonstrates intestinal flora the lesion originates from the bowel, whereas staphylococcal infection comes from the skin; in both cases, however, operative drainage of the pus collection relieves the symptoms. Furthermore, a pre-existing fistula is previously diagnosable (see Sect. 4.3) and in the case of an abscess the development of a fistula is not inevitable. If bacteriological evaluation is desirable, a cotton carrier is contaminated with pus and immediately placed in a transport medium. In suspected gonorrhoea a swab is taken from the orifice of the urethra, the vaginal fornix, and the rectum and immediately carried in a special medium to the laboratory. A possible syphilitic lesion is compressed and the exudate aspirated; it is then examined at once for spirochaetes. Such specimens are highly contagious, making the wearing of gloves advisable.

Stool samples for bacteriological testing are best procured endoscopically. The specimen in a sterile container needs no special care except when amoebiasis is suspected. Examination must be started during the following 3–4 h. Some organisms require specific culturing (e.g. *Campylobacter*, *Clostridium difficile*). Clear information for the bacteriologist is important especially when specific organisms are being sought.

Search for protozoa or worm eggs is possible in a stool sample sent in an unsterile pot to the laboratory by the patient himself. To trap oxyurids a double adhesive tape is stuck on the perianal skin overnight. When the vermicules leave the anus in the early morning they will adhere to the tape.
With the increasing specification of antiviral drugs, virus identification might gain in significance over the carcinoma-predicting value in human papillomavirus (HPV). Specimens (e.g. condylomata acuminata) must be sent either in a special medium or immediately on a wet gauze compress to the laboratory.
Serologic tests to detect antibodies and in the first instance a rising antibody titre identify certain infectious diseases. The greatest concern in coloproctology is human immunodeficiency virus (HIV) infection. In our series 60% of patients suffering from condylomata acuminata are HIV positive. Therefore, every doctor should be aware of the risk of HIV infection in patients (especially those with a sexual transmitted disease) and take precautionary measures for self-protection.

**Appendix.** Symptoms in Coloproctology and Essential Related Diagnoses[a]

| | | |
|---|---|---|
| *Pain* | | |
| Perianal | Continuous | Perianal abscess |
| | | Thrombosed external haemorrhoid |
| | | Herpes simplex analis |
| Anal | During and after defaecation | Anal fissure |
| | | (Intersphincteric abscess) |
| | | (Syphilitic primary sore) |
| | | (Ulcus molle = soft chancre) |
| Anorectal | Paroxysmal, mainly at night | (Proctalgia fugax) |
| | Continuous | Proctitis, cryptitis, papillitis |
| | | Intersphincteric abscess |
| | | Deeply infiltrating carcinoma |
| | | Ulcer in anal canal (e.g. Crohn's disease) |
| | | Prostatitis |
| *Bleeding* | | |
| Blood trace on toilet paper or motion | | Anal fissure |
| | | Maceration of the skin |
| | | (Condylomata acuminata) |
| Blood during/after defaecation | | Internal haemorrhoids |
| | | Adenoma, polyp |
| | | Carcinoma |
| Blood and pus/mucus | | Ulcerative colitis |
| | | Rectal carcinoma |
| | | Acute dysentery |
| Mass bleeding | | Radiation proctitis |
| | | Ulcerative colitis |
| | | Diverticulosis |
| | | Adenoma |

**Appendix** (*continued*)

| | |
|---|---|
| | Carcinoma<br>Haemangioma<br>(Internal haemorrhoids)<br>(Anal fissure) |
| *Discharge* (weeping) | |
| Externally | Perianal dermatitis<br>– Weeping eczema<br>– Mycosis<br>– Skin maceration<br>– Erosions and ulceration |
| Anal | Proctitis<br>Exulcerated carcinoma<br>Villous adenoma<br>Keyhole deformity after surgery |
| Perianal | Fistula |
| *Pruritus ani* | |
| Local causes | Perianal dermatitis<br>– Skin maceration (after abuse of topical steroids)<br>– Eczema<br>– Mycosis<br>Discharge from anus or fistula<br>Insanitary conditions<br>Sexually transmitted disease (e.g. condylomata acuminata) |
| Systemic causes | Psychogenic (idiopathic)<br>Oxyuriasis (mainly in the early morning)<br>Metabolic<br>– Diabetes mellitus<br>– Jaundice<br>Hodgkin's disease<br>Neurodystonia<br>Food allergy<br>Malignancies<br>– Lymphoma<br>(– Paraneoplastic) |
| *Swelling/tumour* | |
| Perianal | Skin tag<br>Thrombosed haemorrhoid<br>Condylomata (acuminata, lata)<br>Abscess<br>Carcinoma<br>Benign tumours |
| Anal canal | Hypertrophic papillae<br>Condylomata acuminata<br>Carcinoma |
| Rectal ampulla | Adenoma/polyp<br>Carcinoma<br>Supralevator abscess<br>Condylomata acuminata<br>(Thrombosed internal haemorrhoid) |

**Appendix** (*continued*)

| | |
|---|---|
| *Prolapse* | Internal haemorrhoids (grades II–IV)<br>Anal mucosa<br>Hypertrophic papilla<br>Rectal prolapse<br>(Polyp/adenoma)<br>(Carcinoma) |
| *Defaecation disorders* | |
| Unsatisfactory evacuation | Proctitis (inflammatory, radiation)<br>Anorectal carcinoma<br>Anorectal prolapse<br>Irritable bowel syndrome<br>Rectocele<br>(Internal haemorrhoids) |
| Urgency | Acute enteritis<br>Crohn's disease<br>Ulcerative colitis<br>Irritable bowel syndrome |
| Hard straining necessary | Constipation<br>Colorectal dysfunction<br>– outlet obstruction (e.g. Hirschsprung's disease, anal dysplasia, levator syndrome)<br>Enterocele |
| Incontinence (cause) | Descending perineum syndrome<br>Sphincter trauma<br>Consistency of motion (diarrhoea)<br>Neurogenic<br>Urgency<br>Loss/irritation of sensitive nerve receptors<br>Psychosomatic<br>Reduction of rectal capacity<br>Rectal prolapse |

[a] Less frequent diseases are shown within parentheses.

## References


1. Buchmann P (1988) Lehrbuch der Proktologie, 2nd edn. Hans Huber, Bern
2. Corman MC (1989) Colon and rectal surgery, 2nd edn. J.B. Lippincott, Philadelphia
3. Marti M-C, Givel J-C (eds) Surgery of anorectal diseases with pre- and post-operative management. Springer, Berlin Heidelberg New York
4. Nicholls J, Glass R (1985) Coloproctology. Diagnosis and outpatient management. Springer, Berlin Heidelberg New York
5. Stein E (1990) Proktologie Lehrbuch und Atlas, 2nd edn. Springer, Berlin Heidelberg New York

# 5 Defaecography: Technique and Radiation Exposure

## 5.1 Technique

W. Brühlmann

### *5.1.1 X-ray Equipment*

Defaecography can be performed using x-ray units with a tilting table, an image intensifier and spot films and/or 100-mm image intensifier photography. A video recorder should be attached to the equipment. Remote control units have the advantages of better access to the patient during defaecography and lower x-ray exposure due to the greater focus–object distance.

### *5.1.2 Patient Seat and Optical Shielding*

The simplest patient seat is a plastic pot placed on the elevated footrest of the x-ray table. However, this is not an optimal solution with respect to patient comfort, stability and hygiene. Hauck has constructed a special seat directly clamped to the x-ray table instead of the footrest (Fig. 5.1).
It consists of a board with a central opening to receive the pot. The pot itself is coated with a disposable plastic bag to receive the faeces. It rests on a ridge with a width of exactly 1 cm, which serves as a caliper for radiographic measurements. A very elaborate seat has been developed by Mahieu (Fig. 5.2): It consists of a stack of air chambers (inner tubes of car tyres) glued together and filled with water to compensate for absorption differences. The expelled faeces are received by a disposable plastic bag.
Some sort of optical shielding is recommended by Goei to allow the patient some privacy during defaecation.

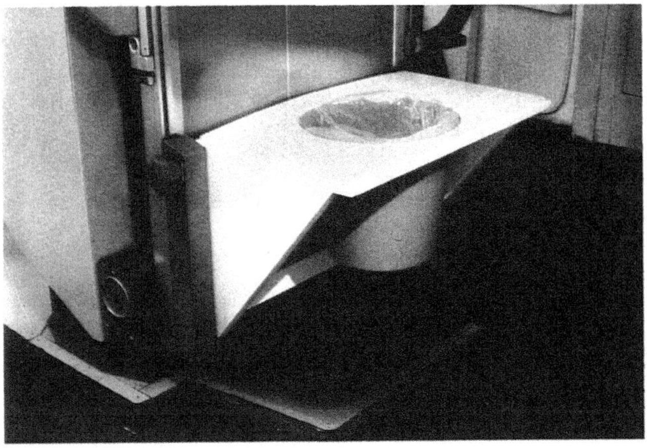

▲

Fig. 5.1. Special seat for defaecography

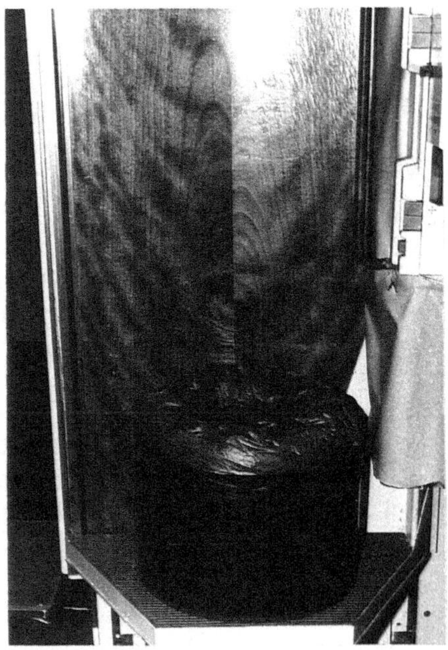

Fig. 5.2. Patient seat designed by Mahieu

### *5.1.3 Compensation for Absorption Differences*

Especially in obese women, there is a large difference in x-ray absorption between the pelvis and the perineum. This can be compensated for by placing a lead foil between the x-ray table and the plastic pot or by the use of graded intensifying screens (Hauck). Both lead filters and intensifying screens should be graded in several steps to avoid sharp edges visible on the film. Intensifying screens should cover a very wide range, with factors from 2 to 16. Screens are, of course, applicable only when employing the conventional spot film technique. A very elegant solution to this problem is the water-filled seat developed by Mahieu, although the water will produce some scattered radiation.

### *5.1.4 Patient Preparation*

The administration of oral laxatives or cleansing enemas is contraindicated, as a sigmoid colon filled with faeces facilitates defaecation. In addition, residual water will lead to the expulsion of liquid rather than semisolid material.

### *5.1.5 Contrast Filling of the Colon*

The lubricant used to insert the rectal tube should not contain local anaesthetics, as a normal sensitivity of the anorectal epithelium is important for defaecation. When a liquid barium sulphate suspension is used, the colon is filled at least to the level of the splenic flexure, to induce the expulsion of faeces.

Mahieu uses a biphasic technique: First, some concentrated high density barium sulphate is introduced into the anorectum to coat the wall. Then, a semisolid suspension thickened with potato starch is introduced.

To make the semisolid contrast medium after Mahieu, 150 ml of a conventional liquid barium sulphate suspension is first diluted in 400 ml of water.

The mixture is heated and gradually mixed with 100 g potato starch, beating with a whisk to prevent clumping, until a smooth thick paste is formed. After cooling, the mixture is filled into a commercially available injection pistol as used for grease or putty (Fig. 5.3).

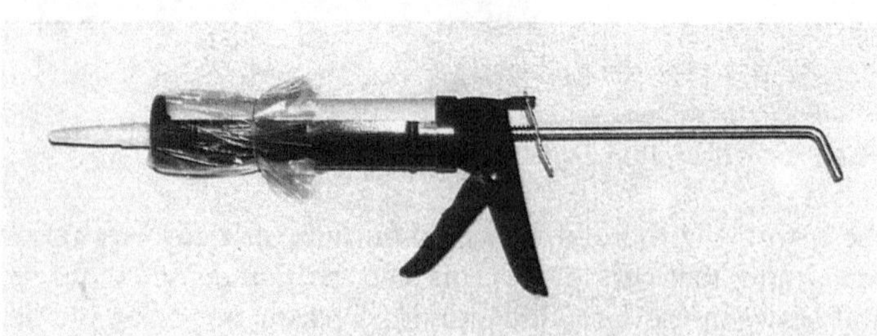

**Fig. 5.3.** Injection pistol for introduction of the semisolid contrast medium

### *5.1.6 Marking Other Structures with Contrast*

The anal orifice should be marked with a thick barium sulphate paste. The vagina is not marked routinely, except by Hauck. It can be opacified with a cotton swab soaked with liquid contrast material, introduced with forceps. Vaginal tampons are not recommended because their stiffness might impede the visualisation of a rectocele. The small bowel is only opacified when there is suspicion of an enterocele, i.e. in patients with a "defaecation block".

### *5.1.7 Imaging During Defaecation*

Critical phases or pathological phenomena can be documented with conventional spot films or 100-mm image intensifier photography. However, documentation of the movements during defaecation by dynamic image acquisition is recommended. Excellent temporal resolution and good image quality are provided by 35-mm cinematography. Serial 100-mm photography has only a limited temporal resolution but provides an excellent image quality. However, both modalities expose the patient to a high amount of radiation (see Sect. 5.2). Video recording combines excellent temporal resolution with relatively low radiation exposure. However, its spatial resolution is not sufficient to depict mucosal detail, which is important in intussusception. Therefore, the best imaging modality available to date seems to be a combination of video recording and single 100-mm frames during critical phases.

### *5.1.8 Additional Manoeuvres*

The patient should be encouraged to watch the fluoroscopic image on the video monitor, as the visual feedback information will facilitate defaecation. After evacuation, elevation of the pelvic floor during a "pinch" or "squeeze" manoeuvre should be documented on video tape.

### *5.1.9 Static Documentation After Evacuation*

After completion of evacuation, spot films during rest and "press" and "pinch" manoeuvres should be exposed. Here, conventional films have the advantage over 100-mm photography that skeletal landmarks such as the symphysis and the coccyx are well visualised, indicating the position of the anorectal angle in relation to the skeleton. However, quantitative measurements are of very limited value (see Chap. 6). Hauck recommends additional films in the anteroposterior projection during rest and during strain, to document lateral outpouchings (see Chap. 16).

## 5.2 Radiation Exposure of the Patient During Defaecography

W. Brühlmann and W. Müller-Duysing

The increasing popularity of defaecography calls for sufficient information about the radiation exposure of the patient due to this diagnostic procedure. Based on in vivo measurements of the exposure at mid-pelvis level with intravaginal detectors, we calculated the ovarian dose for two different imaging modalities (video recording and 35-mm cineradiography).

### *5.2.1 Material and Methods*

All examinations were performed on a conventional x-ray machine with a focus–table distance of 50 cm, equipped with a cine-pulse unit for image intensifier cinematography (Philips Diagnost 66, Super 80 CP generator with automatic kV and mA adjustments for fluoroscopy and cineradiography; cine-pulse time set to 10 ms).

In order to visualise the expulsion of faeces, there was no patient preparation with laxatives or enemas. The colon was filled with a liquid barium sulphate suspension to the level of the left colonic flexure, under fluoroscopic monitoring. The rectosigmoid and descending colon were documented with an average of four 100-mm frames, in the left lateral decubitus position. Evacuation and the elevation of the pelvic floor through pinch manoeures were documented with the patient sitting on a plastic pot placed on the footrest of the x-ray table. After evacuation, a total of three x-rays were performed during rest and press and squeeze manoeuvres (left lateral decubitus position, overhead x-ray tube, 35 × 35 cm film format). Dose measurements were performed during the entire procedure in 14 patients for cineradiography and in five patients for video recording. The two imaging protocols used are specified in Table 5.1.

Thermoluminescent dosimeters were applied to the skin surface of the pelvis on the tube side and on the image intensifier side, and within the vagina, wrapped within a vaginal tampon. The pelvic diameter at the trochanter

**Table 5.1.** Imaging protocols used for defaecography

| | Protocol I | Protocol II |
|---|---|---|
| Filling phase | Fluoroscopy 100-mm frames [4] | Fluoroscopy 100-mm frames [4] |
| Defaecation | 35-mm cinematography 25 frames per second 11.6 ± 5.3 m; 26 ± 12 s | Video recording 38 ± 16.4 s |
| Following evacuation | 35 × 35 cm overhead films [3] | 35 × 35 cm overhead films [3] |

level was measured with a pair of compasses. The average kilovoltages for fluoroscopy (video recording) and cinematography were 100 and 120 kV, respectively. The position of the ovaries was assumed to be 4 cm from the vagina, to each side. The ovarian doses were calculated using published depth dose tables [1].

### 5.2.2 *Results*

The averages of the doses measured on the skin surface on the tube side and within the vagina and the doses calculated for the ovaries are given in Table 5.2.

The mean age of the patients was 52 ± 14 years, with a range of 18–79 years. Twenty-one percent of the patients were women under 40 years of age.

### 5.2.3 *Discussion*

Defaecography or evacuation proctography is a valuable diagnostic tool utilised with increasing frequency. Most patients referred to the radiologist for defaecography are women, with a considerable proportion still at a child-bearing age. Thus, the possibility that defaecography will produce genetic damage is an important consideration. However, information about the radiation exposure through defaecography is sparse.

Since defaecation is a dynamic process, some sort of dynamic image recording is mandatory. There are three possible means of achieving this goal:

1. *100-mm image intensifier photography* with frequent single shots or with serial technique is a semidynamic means of image recording, with an excellent image quality but rather low temporal resolution. Goei and Kemerink [2] have performed dose measurements with this technique and have published a mean ovarian dose of 15 ± 5 mSv for an average of 14 ± 6 100-mm frames. The effective surface area of the image on 100-mm film and, correspondingly, the amount of radiation per frame are

**Table 5.2.** Radiation exposure during defaecography (in mSv)

| | Protocol I | Protocol II |
|---|---|---|
| Skin surface on tube side | 512 ± 327 | 86 ± 35 |
| Vagina | 31 ± 18 | 4 ± 1 |
| Ovary on tube side | 62 ± 36 | 9 ± 3 |
| Ovary on film side | 16 ± 9 | 2 ± 1 |

18 times greater than with 35-mm film. Thus, 14 100-mm frames correspond to approximately 10 s of 35-mm filming at 25 frames per second. Thus, the mean ovarian dose of 15 mSv for 14 frames corresponds very well with the dose of 31 mSv at mid-pelvis that we have measured for 26 s of 35-mm filming. The serial 100-mm technique with one to six frames per second offers still poor temporal resolution. In addition, radiation exposure to the patient would be even higher than with cineradiography. For instance, the serial 100-mm technique with two frames per second delivers 1.5 times the dose produced by cineradiography with 25 frames per second.

2. *Video recording* has the disadvantage of a considerably poorer image quality. Sometimes, additional 100 mm frames will therefore be necessary. For the entire procedure, using only video recording during the evacuation phase, we have measured doses of 9 mSv for the ovary proximal to the x-ray tube and 2 mSv for the distal ovary. This compares favourably with the mean ovarian doses of 4–16 mSv published for barium contrast examination of the colon [3, 4].
3. *Cineradiography* combines good image quality with excellent temporal resolution. It is excellent for the examination of deglutition disorders [5], where it exposes the patient to moderate doses of radiation (10 mSv to the thyroid gland). However, our measuremeents indicate that, during defaecography, a dose exceeding 60 mSv is delivered to the ovary proximal to the x-ray tube. Moreover, the entrance dose delivered to the skin surface amounts to more than 500 mSv. These x-ray exposures are unacceptably high for a diagnostic procedure applied in some cases to women of child-bearing age. We have, therefore, discontinued the use of cineradiography for this purpose.

### *5.2.4 Summary and Conclusions*

Cineradiography, although combining good image quality with excellent temporal resolution, delivers unacceptably high radiation doses to patients when used for defaecography. It therefore cannot be advocated for that purpose.

The serial 100-mm technique offers excellent image quality but combines the disadvantages of poor temporal resolution and very high radiation exposure.

Video recording exposes the patient to only a moderate amount of radiation. However, due to its limited image quality, pathological phenomena should be documented with 100-mm frames.

Thus, in our opinion, the best available imaging modality for defaecography is a combination of video recording and a limited number of single 100-mm frames to document pathological phenomena.

## References

1. Wachsmann F, Drexler G (1976) Graphs and tables for use in radiology. Springer, Berlin Heidelberg New York
2. Goei R, Kemerink G (1990) Radiation dose in defecography. Radiology 176:137–139
3. Ranniko S, Servomaa A, Ermakoff I et al. (1987) Calculation of the estimated effective dose equivalent (SE) due to x-ray diagnostic examinations: estimate of the SE in Finland. Health Phys 53:31–36
4. Shrimpton PC, Wall BF, Jones DG et al. (1986) Doses to patients from routine diagnostic x-ray examinations in England. Br J Radiol 59:749–758
5. Brühlmann W (1985) Die röntgenkinematographische Untersuchung von Störungen des Schluckaktes. Huber, Bern

# 6 Defaecographic Parameters in Asymptomatic Subjects

R. Goei

In the past 7 years several authors have described normal defaecographic parameters. The earliest defaecographic measurement was reported in 1969 by Hardcastle [1], who studied the size of the resting anorectal angle and cited an average of 82° in normal persons and an increase to more than 130° in patients with severe degrees of the descending perineum syndrome. In 1984 Mahieu et al. [2] published results based on 56 defaecograms which were considered normal and found a mean value of 91.96° ± 1.52° at rest and an increase to a mean value of 136.76° ± 1.51° during straining. He measured an increase in the anorectal angle in all subjects from rest to straining. No changes in the shape of the rectal wall during evacuation of rectal contents were reported in this study.

In 1987 Skomorowska [3] measured the anorectal angle in 80 asymptomatic subjects aged 27–74 years and found mean values at rest of 108° in women and 127° in men. The authors stated that the values of the anorectal angles in men and women differed significantly. Changes in the shape of the rectal wall during defaecation were not mentioned in this study either.

In 1988 Bartram et al. [4] reported the measurements from the defaecograms of ten males and ten females without defaecation disorders and stated that the anorectal angle was 115° ± 17° at rest and 118° ± 16° during evacuation as measured along the central axis of the lumen, compared with 94° ± 19° and 118° ± 16° using the posterior wall of the rectum. The authors reported small folds during straining, mainly in the posterior wall of the rectum, and some bulging of the anterior wall to form shallow rectoceles.

The differences in the measurements reported by the above-mentioned authors were probably due to the differences in defining the anorectal angle, in the technique of defaecography (including the consistency of the contrast medium) and in the age of the studied subjects.

## 6.1 Study Design and Results

To provide a baseline for the study of abnormal function in our patient group, we conducted a study in 1987 through 1988 in 32 individuals without defaecation disorders who had been referred for barium enema study [5].

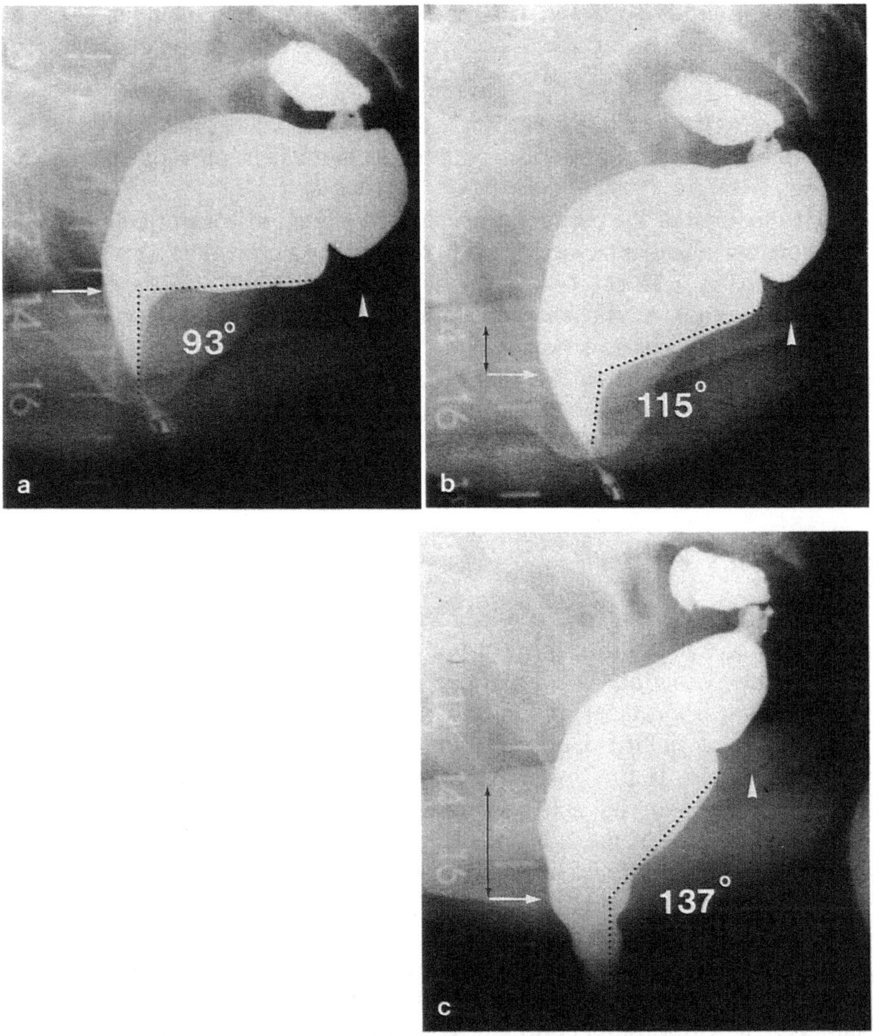


**Fig. 6.1a–c.** Defaecographic parameters. **a** During squeezing the anorectal angle measured 93° (*dotted line*) and the anorectal junction (*arrow*) was near the level of the tip of the coccyx (*arrowhead*). **b** At rest the anorectal angle was 115° (*dotted line*) and the anorectal junction (*arrow*) was 1.7 cm (1.2 units of the ruler ×1.4 magnification factor) (*double-ended arrow*) below the tip of the coccyx (*arrowhead*). **c** During straining the anorectal angle (*dotted line*) widened to 137° and the anorectal junction (*arrow*) descended to 4.2 cm (3.0 units of the ruler ×1.4 magnification factor) (*double-ended arrow*) below the tip of the coccyx (*arrowhead*)

This patient group consisted of 19 males and 13 females ranging in age from 41 to 71 years. During the successive stages of defaecation the following parameters were considered:

1. The anorectal angle, i.e. the angle between the axis of the anal canal and a line along the posterior border of the distal part of the rectum (Fig. 6.1a)
2. The position of the anorectal junction (the point at which the lines of the anorectal angle intersected) with respect to the level of the tip of the coccyx (Fig. 6.1b,c)
3. The elevation of the anorectal junction from rest to squeezing and its descent from rest to straining
4. The maximal width of the anal canal
5. The completeness of rectal emptying
6. The morphological changes of the rectal wall (Fig. 6.4)

### *6.1.1 The Anorectal Angle*

Although the method of measurement was uniform, wide interobserver variability was found in respect of the anorectal angle (Fig. 6.2). Figure 6.3 shows wide variation in all parameters pertaining to anorectal motility during the various stages of defaecation in asymptomatic persons.

This study also yielded data conflicting with those reported in the literature. Various authors [e.g. 2, 4] have stated that the anorectal angle widens during straining in all subjects; in our study, however, the angulation decreased in 16% of the subjects (Table 6.1). This indicates non-relaxation of the pelvic floor muscles during defaecation straining. Similar observations were made by Shorvon et al. [6], who observed a decrease in the anorectal angle during straining in 6 of 17 men and 4 of 15 women.

In our study, during squeezing there was a decrease in the anorectal angle in 30 of the 32 subjects as measured by two observers. In the remaining two subjects, the two observers disagreed on whether there was an increase or a decrease in the anorectal angle (Table 6.1). Shorvon et al. [6] also described

**Table 6.1.** Changes in the anorectal angle (ARA) during defaecation in 32 asymptomatic subjects[a]

| Stage of defaecation | Mean ± SD (degrees) | Range (degrees) | Increased ARA | Decreased ARA | Kappa value |
|---|---|---|---|---|---|
| From rest to straining | 17 ± 24 | −30 to 80 | 27 | 5 | 0.57 |
| From rest to squeezing | 23 ± 19 | −4 to 69 | 2 | 30 | −0.30 |

[a] Negative values denote decrease in ARA. Positive values denote increase in ARA.

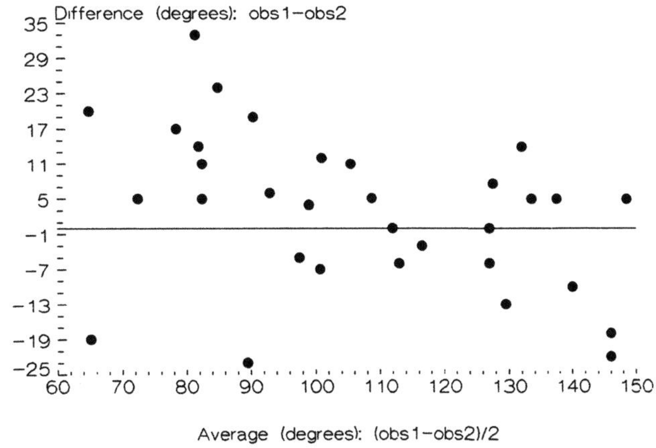


**Fig. 6.2.** Difference against mean for the data of the anorectal angle at rest, measured by observer 1 (*obs1*) and observer 2 (*obs2*)

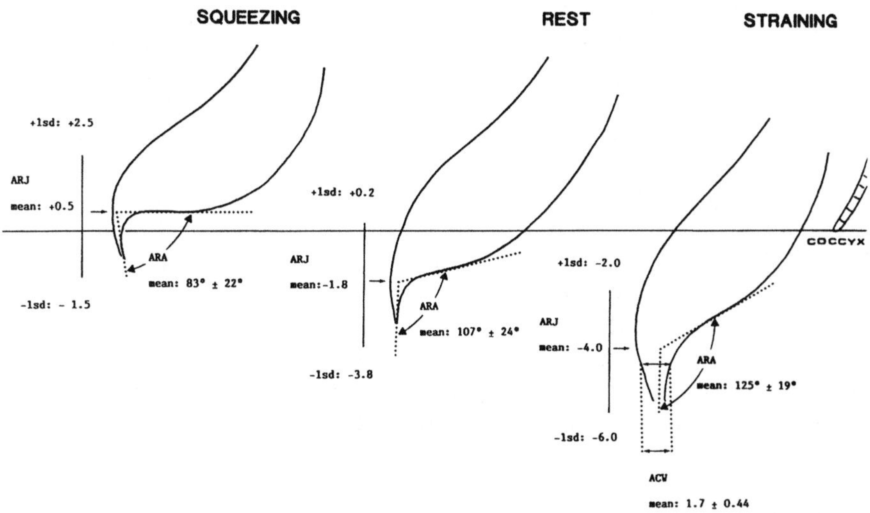


**Fig. 6.3.** Position of the anorectal junction (*ARJ*) with respect to the tip of the coccyx (in cm) and values of the anorectal angle (*ARA*) and anal canal width (*ACW*) during the successive stages of defaecation. All values were the averages of the two observers and thus represented the best estimates of the true values

**Table 6.2.** Changes in excursion of the anorectal junction (ARJ) during defaecation in 32 asymptomatic subjects[a]

| Stage of defaecation | Mean ± SD (cm) | Range (cm) | ARJ descent | ARJ ascent | Kappa value |
|---|---|---|---|---|---|
| From rest to straining | 2.4 ± 1.8 | −7.5 to 0.1 | 29 | 3 | 0.47 |
| From rest to squeezing | 2.3 ± 1.4 | 0.1–5.4 | 0 | 32 | 0 |

[a] Negative values denote descent of ARJ. Positive values denote ascent of ARJ.

subjects in whom there was no change or even an increase in the angulation during squeezing.

### *6.1.2 The Anorectal Junction and Its Movements*

Apart from the changes in the anorectal angle, another parameter of anorectal motility is the changes in the position of the anorectal junction. Similar to the anorectal angle, the position of the anorectal junction showed wide variability during the successive stages of defaecation, a fact confirmed by the study of Shorvon et al. [6]. From rest to squeezing there was an ascent of the anorectal junction in all cases, while from rest to straining there was a descent in 29 cases and an ascent in three (Table 6.2). Shorvon et al. [6] reported that during squeezing all subjects raised the pelvic floor and that on defaectation the pelvic floor descended in 98% of subjects. There was also a wide variation in perineal floor movement, from 18 to 57 mm in men and from 7 to 59 mm in women, with no significant differences between the sexes.

Although Skomorowska et al. [3] showed significant sex differences in the anorectal angle and perineal descent, this finding was not confirmed by the study of Shorvon et al. [6] or by our study [5] (Table 6.3).

### *6.1.3 The Anal Canal*

In our study [5] the anal canal was closed in all subjects during squeezing and at rest. During maximal straining, however, the anal canal opened in all subjects. In the study of Shorvon et al. [6], 8% of the healthy subjects (without complaints of faecal incontinence) had either an open or a partly open anal canal at rest.

**Table 6.3.** Differences in defaecographic measurements between sexes[a]

| Measurements | Men ($n$ = 19) | Women ($n$ = 13) |
|---|---|---|
| *Anorectal angle (degrees)* | | |
| At squeezing | 81 ± 23 | 86 ± 20 |
| At rest | 104 ± 25 | 112 ± 23 |
| At straining | 122 ± 22 | 129 ± 11 |
| From rest to straining | 16 ± 25 | 19 ± 24 |
| From rest to squeezing | 22 ± 20 | 25 ± 19 |
| *Anorectal junction (cm)* | | |
| At squeezing | 0.7 ± 2.1[b] | 0.3 ± 1.8[b] |
| At rest | −1.7 ± 2.4[c] | −1.8 ± 1.8[c] |
| At straining | −3.6 ± 2.5[c] | −4.5 ± 1.5[c] |
| From rest to straining | 2.4 ± 1.8 | 2.6 ± 2.0 |
| From rest to squeezing | 2.5 ± 1.5 | 2.1 ± 1.3 |
| *Anal canal width (cm)* | | |
| At squeezing | 0 | 0 |
| At rest | 0 | 0 |
| At straining | 1.7 ± 0.4 | 1.8 ± 0.4 |

[a] Numbers represent mean ± SD. The Wilcoxon rank sum test for independent samples was used for analysis. All $P$ values were insignificant.
[b] Position above the level of the tip of the coccyx.
[c] Position below the level of the tip of the coccyx.

### *6.1.4 Rectal Emptying*

Although the 32 subjects were instructed to evacuate the contrast medium completely, 17 who did not have a sensation of incomplete evacuation showed residual contrast material in the rectum. Probably this was caused by an abolished sensation of rectal fullness after most of the rectal contents had been expelled, so that these subjects had no need to defaecate any further.

Shorvon et al. [6] found it difficult to measure rectal emptying objectively. They stated that it is difficult to control factors influencing rectal emptying, such as barium reflux to the sigmoid colon, the degree of rectal distension, the consistency of the contrast medium and the straining effort of the subject. There were no data on rectal emptying from these authors or from other studies.

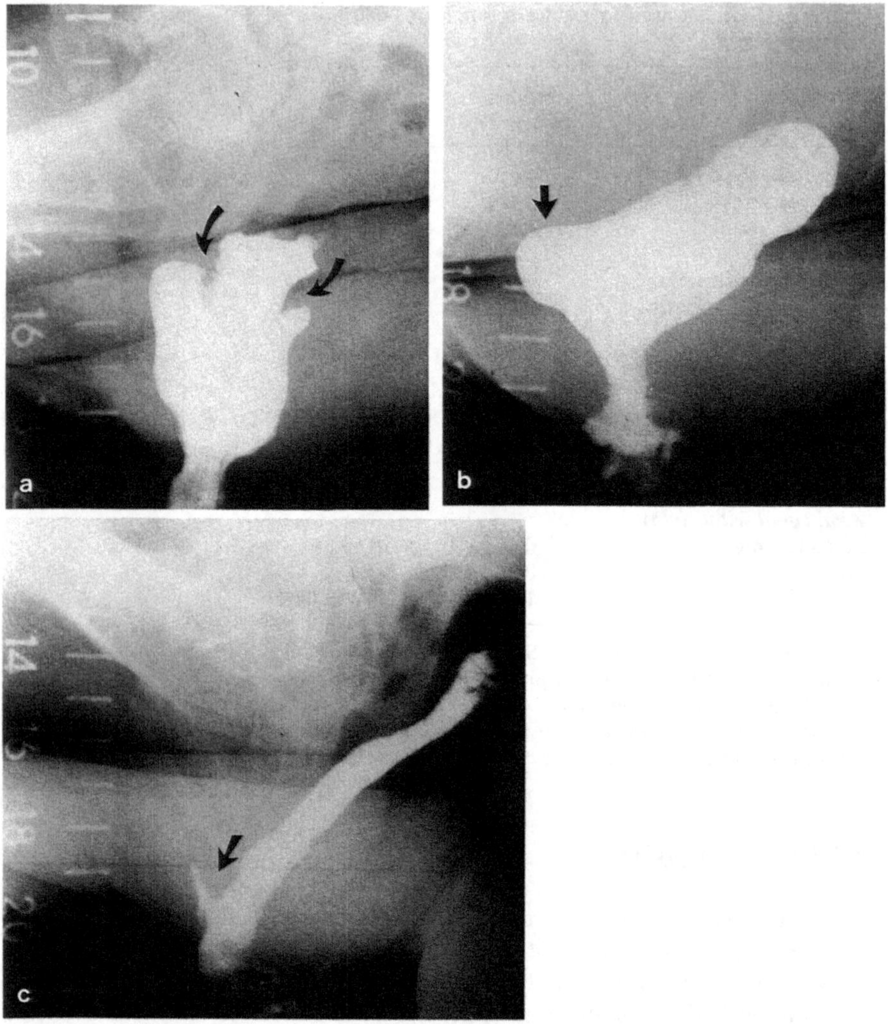


**Fig. 6.4a–c.** Defaecograms of rectal wall abnormalities during straining. **a** Annular intussusception of the proximal rectal wall into its distal lumen (*arrows*). **b** Outpocketing of the anterior rectal wall forms a rectocele (*arrow*). **c** Slight infolding at the anterior rectal wall represents a mucosal prolapse (*arrow*)

### *6.1.5 Rectal Wall Abnormalities*

In our study [5] rectal wall abnormalities, such as intussusception, rectocele and mucosal prolapse, were present in 10 of 32 patients (Table 6.4, Fig. 6.4). It is remarkable that changes in the shape of the rectal wall during straining were not mentioned in several studies on anorectal motility in healthy subjects. Bartram et al. [4] and Shorvon et al. [6], however, described

**Table 6.4.** Classification of defaecograms

| | Control subjects ($n$ = 32) | Patients ($n$ = 32) | Total consecutive patients ($n$ = 155) |
|---|---|---|---|
| Normal | 17 (53%) | 12 (38%) | 32 (21%) |
| Abnormal | 10 (32%) | 19 (59%) | 113 (73%) |
| Equivocal | 5 (16%) | 1 (3%) | 10 (6%) |

anatomical changes of the anorectum during defaecation straining, such as intussusception, mucosal prolapse, rectocele and enterocele.

## 6.2 Differences in Measurements Between Asymptomatic and Symptomatic Subjects

It is obvious from several studies that there is wide variation in anorectal function in asymptomatic subjects, and that abnormalities of the rectal wall during defaecation straining occur in approximately 30%. Therefore, the question can be raised as to whether and, if so, to what extent anorectal function in patients with defaecation disorders differs from that in asymptomatic subjects.

To answer this question a comparative study [7] of several defaecographic parameters was conducted in a group of patients with defaecation disorders and a control group of asymptomatic subjects. The results showed that the radiological measurements of anorectal function in the patients with defaecation disorders, whether the patients were constipated or incontinent, did not differ significantly from the measurements in the asymptomatic subjects (Table 6.5).

These findings indicate that defaecographic measurements cannot be regarded as reliable indicators of the complex physiological condition of the pelvic floor muscles. Although the width of the anal canal during squeezing and rest differed significantly between the patients and the control subjects, during straining the differences were not significant, which suggests that these observations were probably of no clinical consequence.

The results from the aforementioned study were confirmed by Womack et al. [8], who reported no significant differences in the anorectal angle at defaecation straining between constipated subjects and control subjects. Bartolo et al. [9] found no significant differences in the anorectal angle between continent and incontinent patients.

Table 6.6 shows the findings at defaecography in our control group and the patient group. From this it is clear that rectal wall abnormalities were present in a large proportion of the patients. Rectal wall intussusception, rectocele, the spastic pelvic floor syndrome and the solitary rectal ulcer syndrome were the most frequent findings at defaecography in the patients.

**Table 6.5.** Measurements of anorectal motility in 32 control subjects and 32 patients[a]

| Variable[b] | Control subjects ($n$ = 32) | Symptomatic patients | | $P$[c] | Significant[d] |
|---|---|---|---|---|---|
| | | Constipation ($n$ = 19) | Incontinence ($n$ = 13) | | |
| *Squeezing* | | | | | |
| ARA | 83° ± 22° | 80° ± 23° | 84° ± 33° | 0.90 | No |
| ARJ | 0.5 ± 2.0 | 0.2 ± 2.1 | 0.7 ± 2.3 | 0.74 | No |
| ACW | 0 | 0.20 ± 0.28 | 0.28 ± 0.46 | 0.003 | Yes |
| *Rest* | | | | | |
| ARA | 107° ± 24° | 103° ± 22° | 102° ± 30° | 0.70 | No |
| ARJ | −1.8 ± 2.0 | −2.3 ± 1.8 | −1.5 ± 2.5 | 0.42 | No |
| ACW | 0 | 0.27 ± 0.53 | 0.47 ± 0.64 | 0.0002 | Yes |
| *Straining* | | | | | |
| ARA | 125° ± 19° | 121° ± 30° | 128° ± 41° | 0.56 | No |
| ARJ | −4.0 ± 2.0 | −4.0 ± 2.4 | −3.6 ± 3.3 | 0.96 | No |
| ACW | 1.7 ± 0.44 | 1.07 ± 0.53 | 1.46 ± 0.71 | 0.28 | No |
| *ARA* | | | | | |
| Rest → straining | 17° ± 24° | 19° ± 25° | 26° ± 27° | 0.52 | No |
| Rest → squeezing | 23° ± 19° | 22° ± 13° | 18° ± 16° | 0.72 | No |
| *ARJ* | | | | | |
| Rest → straining | 2.4 ± 1.8 | 1.7 ± 1.4 | 2.1 ± 1.8 | 0.44 | No |
| Rest → squeezing | 2.3 ± 1.4 | 2.1 ± 1.5 | 2.2 ± 1.4 | 0.87 | No |

ARA, anorectal angle; ARJ, anorectal junction; ACW, anal canal width.
[a] Measurements are reported as mean ± SD.
[b] "Anorectal junction" indicates position of junction relative to the tip of the coccyx.
[c] Wilcoxon rank sum for independent samples.
[d] Level of significance, $P < 0.01$.

The main role of defaecography is to document these abnormalities as a guide to surgical therapy (if any such therapy is required).

## 6.3 Conclusions

1. There is wide interobserver variation in the measurements of defaecographic parameters.
2. There is also wide variation in the patterns of anorectal function among healthy individuals.
3. Although the anatomy of the male and female pelvis differs, there are no differences between the sexes in the motility of the anorectum.
4. Radiological measurements of anorectal function in patients with defaecation disorders, whether the patients are constipated or incontinent, do not differ from measurements in asymptomatic subjects.

**Table 6.6.** Findings at defaecography

| Findings | Control subjects ($n$ = 32) | Patients ($n$ = 32) | Total consecutive patients ($n$ = 155) |
|---|---|---|---|
| Intussusception | 4 (13%) | 7 (22%) | 29 (19%) |
| Spastic pelvic floor syndrome | 0[a] | 6 (19%) | 23 (15%) |
| Solitary rectal ulcer | 0 | 2 (6%) | 20 (13%) |
| Intussusception + rectocele | 0 | 1 (3%) | 11 (7%) |
| Rectocele | 3 (9%) | 0 | 9 (6%) |
| Prolapse | 0 | 1 (3%) | 4 (3%) |
| Mucosal prolapse or intussusception | 3 (9%) | 2 (6%) | 6 (4%) |
| (possible) | 0 | 0 | 3 (2%) |
| Descending perineum syndrome | 0 | 0 | 1 (0.6%) |
| Rectovaginal fistula | 5 (16%) | 1 (3%) | 10 (6%) |
| Equivocal | 0 | 0 | 7 (5%) |
| Unexplained inability to evacuate | | | |
| Total | 15 (47%) | 20 (63%) | 123 (80%) |

[a] Five subjects showed a decrease in the anorectal angle during straining but evacuated most of the rectal contents.

It is questionable whether measurements on defaecograms reflect the physiology of the anorectum. Therefore these measurements should be interpreted with caution and should not be used as the main criteria for treatment.

5. Quite a high proportion of healthy individuals show abnormalities in the shape of the anorectal wall during defaecation straining, such as intussusception, mucosal prolapse, rectocele and enterocele. Apparently these changes do not necessarily cause symptoms. Whether they will progress and ultimately give rise to a clinically mainfested disorder needs further investigation.
6. The main application of defaecography is for the detection of anatomical abnormalities as a possible cause of defaecation disorders.

## References

1. Hardcastle JD (1969) The descending perineum syndrome. Practitioner 203:612–619
2. Mahieu P, Pringot J, Bodart P (1984) Defecography: I. Description of a new procedure and results in normal patients. Gastrointest Radiol 9:247–251
3. Skomorowska E, Henrichsen S, Christiansen J, Hegedüs V (1987) Acta Radiol 28:559–562
4. Bartram CI, Turnbull GK, Lennard-Jones JE (1988) Evacuation proctography: an investigation of rectal expulsion in 20 subjects without defecatory disturbance. Gastrointest Radiol 13:72–80

5. Goei R, van Engelshoven J, Schouten H, Baeten C, Stassen C (1989) Anorectal function: defecographic measurement in asymptomatic subjects. Radiology 173:137–141
6. Shorvon PJ, McHugh S, Diamant NE, Somers S, Stevenson GW (1989) Defecography in normal volunteers: results and implications. Gut 30:1737–1749
7. Goei R (1990) Anorectal function in patients with defecation disorders and asymptomatic subjects. Evaluation with defecography. Radiology 174:121–123
8. Womack NR, Williams NS, Holmfield JHM, Morrison JFB, Simpkins KC (1985) New method for the dynamic assessment of anorectal function in constipation. Br J Surg 72:994–998
9. Bartolo DCC, Read NW, Jarratt JA, Read MG, Donnelly TC, Johnson AG (1983) Differences in anal sphincter function and clinical presentation in patients with pelvic floor descent. Gastroenterology 85:68–75

# 7 Indications for Defaecography

The following list reflects the consensus of the participants in the workshop that formed the basis for this book with respect to the indications for defaecography *in adults*:

| | |
|---|---|
| *Symptoms* | |
| – Feeling of incomplete evacuation | + |
| – Blocked evacuation | + |
| – Heaviness, "perineal mass" | + |
| – Heavy straining during defaecation | + |
| – Need for digital assistance | + |
| – Chronic constipation | (+) |
| – Faecal incontinence | – |
| *Objective findings* | |
| – Mucosal lesion of anterior rectal wall | + |
| – Rectocele of more than 2 cm on palpation | + |
| – Slow transit through distal part of colon | + |
| – Intussusception as seen by rectoscopy | (+) |
| *Suspicion of* | |
| – Occult intussusception | + |
| – Occult prolapse | + |
| – Enterocele | + |

## 7.1 Indications in Adults: The Physician's View

A. Rühl and J.F. Erckenbrecht

Defaecography is a dynamic method of radiological investigation for the documentation of functional and morphological changes of the anorectum and pelvic floor during defaecation. Therefore, defaecography renders information on defaecation disorders complementary to that provided by the case history, clinical examination, endoscopy, anorectal manometry, electrophysiological investigation, transit time measurement and endosonography [1–4].

**Table 7.1.** Diagnostic procedures in anorectal diseases

| Method | Inconvenience for patient | Expense of procedure | Relevance for treatment decisions |
|---|---|---|---|
| History | (+) | 0 | +++ |
| Clinical examination | (+) | 0 | +++ |
| Endoscopy | + | ++ | ++ |
| Manometry | ++ | +++ | ++ |
| EMG | +++ | +++ | ++ |
| Endosonography | ++ | +++ | + |
| Defaecography | ++ | ++ | ++ |
| CT/MRI | + | +++ | + |

The defaecation disorders investigated by means of defaecography are (a) constipation/feeling of incomplete evaculation and (b) faecal incontinence/ faecal soiling. Furthermore, defaecography should be performed if a patient presents with symptoms compatible with organic anorectal disease when endoscopy is normal or shows a solitary rectal ulcer [4, 5]. Such symptoms are anorectal pain, transanal bleeding, transanal secretions, mucous discharge and pruritus ani.

Among the different procedures commonly employed in anorectal investigation, defaecography entails as much inconvenience for the patient as anorectal manometry or endosonography, while it is better tolerated than anorectal electromyography. Costs are comparable to those of endoscopy, while the other diagnostic procedures for anorectal disorders are more expensive (Table 7.1).

The technique of defaecography and defaecographic parameters are discussed in Chaps. 5 and 6.

### *7.1.1 Constipation/Feeling of Incomplete Evacuation*

Patients with constipation can be differentiated into two major groups. In the first group, colonic motility is impaired and transit time is prolonged in all colonic segments ("*colonic inertia: slow transit constipation*"). The second group is characterised by normal colonic transit up to the rectosigmoid, where transit time is prolonged. In this group, defaecation disorders can be detected: the patient is not able to evacuate properly ("*outlet obstruction*").

Outlet obstruction can be caused by three different mechanisms: insufficient relaxation of the internal anal sphincter (Hirschsprung's disease), improper contraction of the external anal sphincter ("anismus") or mechanical obstruction occurring in the process of defaecation (caused by, for example, intussusception, rectocele or enterocele).

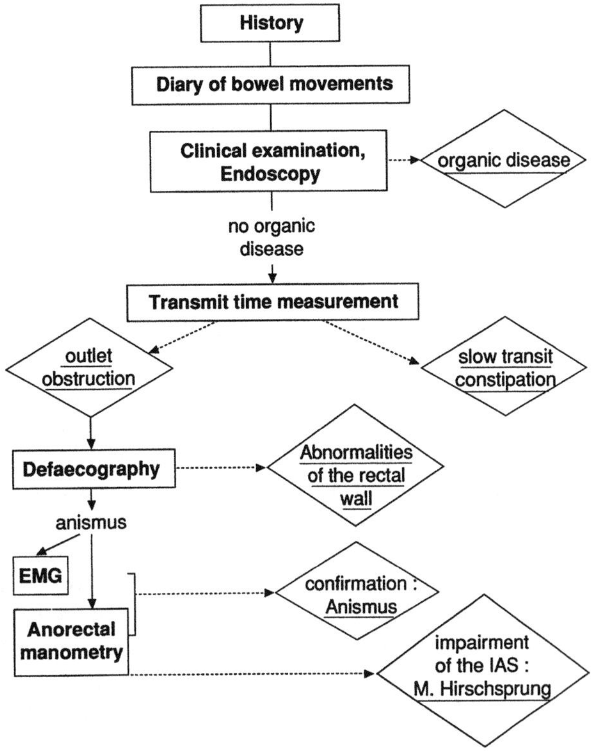


**Fig. 7.1.** Application of diagnostic methods in constipation. Diagnoses are *underlined* and enclosed within *lozenges*. The *broken arrows* indicate pathological findings. *IAS*, internal anal sphincter

Differentiation between slow transit constipation and outlet obstruction can be achieved by means of segmental colonic transit time measurement [6, 7] (cf. Chap. 13), anorectal manometry, anal electromyography (cf. Chap. 14) and defaecography (Fig. 7.1).

Defaecographic findings in constipation/feeling of incomplete evacuation may reveal the cause of outlet obstruction:

1. *Rectal intussusception and rectal prolapse* (cf. Chap. 15). Intussusceptions are infoldings of the rectal wall with a length of more than 1 cm. Intussusceptions appear at the end of defaecation. Therefore, most intussusceptions can only be demonstrated defaecographically. If intussusceptions become more pronounced or even result in a complete rectal prolapse [2, 8, 9], they can obturate the rectal lumen during defaecation and thus cause mechanical outlet obstruction.
2. *Rectoceles* (cf. Chap. 16). Rectoceles are outpocketings of the rectal wall with a diameter of more than 1 cm. During defaecation, parts of the faeces may be sequestered into a rectocele, which subsequently obturates

the lumen of the anorectum. As rectoceles appear only during defaecation, defaecography is the investigation of choice to demonstrate the existence of this anomaly of the rectal wall. However, rectoceles are common defaecographic findings and are mostly without clinical significance [8, 10].

3. *Enteroceles* (cf. Chap. 17). Enteroceles may cause an extraluminal obstruction of the anorectum when intra-abdominal pressure rises during defaecation. Enteroceles are rarely the underlying reason for an outlet obstruction.
4. *Anismus/spastic pelvic floor syndrome* (cf. Chaps. 18 and 20). In *anismus*, the physiological relaxation of the pelvic floor musculature during defaecation is impaired [11, 12]. Instead of relaxing the puborectalis muscle and the external anal sphincter, patients contract these muscles during their efforts to evacuate and thus are unable to defaecate properly. During straining efforts, defaecography shows no widening of the anorectal angle or even an accentuation of the impression of the puborectalis muscle; the pelvic floor does not descend and the anal canal remains closed. The patient may be completely unable to expel the contrast medium. To confirm the diagnosis of anismus, anorectal manometry and electromyography should be performed. Whether anismus is a distinct clinical syndrome or an artefact due to the embarrassing investigational situation is still under discussion [7, 11–16]. Some investigators have been able to show therapeutic improvement when the improper contractions of the pelvic floor muscles are treated with anorectal biofeedback training [7, 13, 17].
5. *Descending perineum syndrome* (Chap. 19). During straining, the pelvic floor descends physiologically while the pelvic floor musculature relaxes. In the descending perineum syndrome, the extent of descent of the pelvic floor is beyond the range in normals (>2–3 cm; [18, 19]). The descending perineum syndrome can be associated with constipation or faecal incontinence. In the case of constipation, the descending perineum syndrome is nowadays supposed to be the consequence of chronic straining at stools (a common finding in constipation) rather than an independent pathogenetic mechanism. Chronic straining at stools causes chronic pudendal neuropathy [20, 21]. The extent of the perineal descent in constipation thus indicates the degree of damage of the pudendal and perineal nerves and may lead to neurogenic ("idiopathic") incontinence [22, 23].

### *7.1.2 Faecal Incontinence/Faecal Soiling*

An aetiological classification of faecal incontinence discriminates three forms:

1. *"Idiopathic faecal incontinence"* without other symptoms or history of anal damage is the most common form of faecal incontinence. It is caused by neuropathy of the pudendal and/or perineal nerves [22, 24, 25].

2. *Myogenic incontinence* may be caused by trauma (proctological surgery, obstertric trauma, accidents), inflammation, ischaemia or myopathies. Faecal incontinence because of congenital anorectal malformations usually shows features of both neurogenic damage and muscle defects.
3. The cause of *functional incontinence* is located outside of the anorectum, as, for example, in diarrhoea, where the normal continence mechanisms are overwhelmed by the challenge of masses of loose stools.

Diagnostic procedures to clarify the aetiology of faecal incontinence/faecal soiling are anorectal manometry, electrophysiological studies (Chap. 14), endosonography of the anorectum (Chap. 2) and defaecography. Each diagnostic procedure renders complementary information (Fig. 7.2).
Defaecography is not feasible in patients with major incontinence (frequent involuntary loss of formed stools), as these patients with spontaneous leakage of barium are often totally unable to retain the contrast medium. Furthermore, clear defaecographic characteristics of faecal incontinence in these patients have not yet been established. However, if patients complain of minor incontinence or faecal soiling, defaecography may be able to reveal an underlying abnormality not detectably by other methods.
Facultative defaecographic findings in faecal incontinence/faecal soiling are:

1. *Rectal intussusception and rectoceles*. Faecal soiling may be caused by rectoceles and/or intussusceptions when parts of the rectosigmoid are occluded during straining. Faeces retained in these parts of the intestine can flow out of the anal canal when the occlusion dissolves at rest.
2. *Rectal prolapse*. Often, but not always, rectal prolapse is associated with faecal incontinence. Whether there is a cause-effect relationship between rectal prolapse and faecal incontinence or whether there is a common aetiological origin is not yet established [22, 26–28].
3. *Anismus/spastic pelvic floor syndrome*. Overflow incontinence occurring as faecal soiling is one of the most distressing complications of faecal impaction. Patients with faecal impaction and faecal incontinence have impaired anorectal sensations. Furthermore, the rectoanal inhibitory reflex is elicited by smaller distension volumes than in normal controls [29]. In patients with the spastic pelvic floor syndrome, retention of stools in the rectum may be the cause of faecal impaction and thus of overflow incontinence. In these patients, outlet obstruction as the hidden cause of faecal soiling/incontinence can be revealed with the help of defaecography.
4. *Descending perineum syndrome*. As already mentioned, the descending perineum syndrome can be associated with constipation or faecal incontinence. The degree of perineal descent indicates the degree of damage of the innervation of the pelvic floor [18], while pudendal and perineal neuropathies are related with faecal incontinence [22–26]. Thus, perineal descent may predict neurogenic ("idiopathic") incontinence.
5. *Widening of the anorectal angle*. If incontinence is a consequence of damage to the pelvic floor innervation ("idiopathic", "primary", neuro-

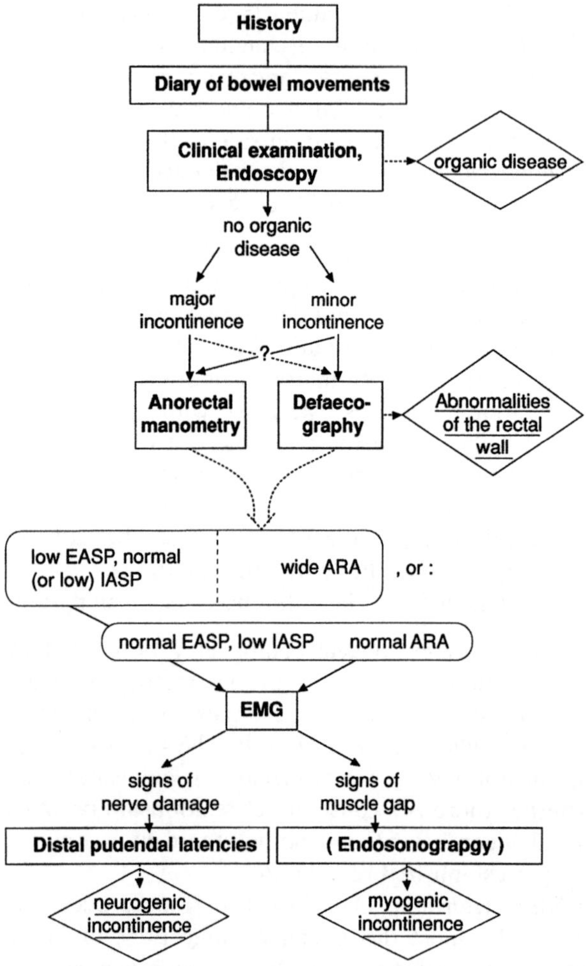


**Fig. 7.2.** Application of diagnostic methods in faecal incontinence. Diagnoses are *underlined* and enclosed within *lozenges*. The *broken arrows* indicate pathological findings. *EASP*, pressure of the external anal sphincter; *IASP*, pressure of the internal anal sphincter; *ARA*, anorectal angle

genic faecal incontinence), in most cases not only the external anal sphincter but also the puborectal is muscle is involved [30]. In defaecography, the degree of anorectal angulation is determined by the strength of the puborectalis muscle. Therefore, in neurogenic incontinence the anorectal angle tends to be wider than in normal persons or patients who are incontinent because of muscle rupture or other muscle defects. Furthermore, the decrease in the anorectal angle during contraction is less marked than in normal controls. However, defaecographic evaluation of a pathologically widened anorectal angle may be difficult, as the range of values in normal males is too great to permit clear cut-off values to be set down for normal and pathological findings [19], and there is a large overlap between "normal" and "pathological" values of the anorectal angle (cf. Chap. 6).

### *7.1.3 Solitary Rectal Ulcer Syndrome*

Usually, the diagnosis of a solitary rectal ulcer is established endoscopically (cf. Chap. 11), but defaecography may help to establish the a etiology of a solitary rectal ulcer syndrome. The most common causes of a solitary rectal ulcer are intussusceptions and complete rectal prolapse with the ulcer located at the tip of the protruding mucosa [4, 5, 9]. If a solitary rectal ulcer cannot be healed conservatively and defaecography shows an ulcer-related rectal intussusception or rectal prolapse, surgical therapy is indicated. Good results have been reported after surgical intervention in solitary rectal ulcers [5, 31].

### *7.1.4 Conclusions*

Defaecography is indicated if symptoms of anorectal disorders raise suspicion of changes in the rectal shape during defaecation. No other method is able to demonstrate the configuration of the rectal wall under functional circumstances as clearly as defaecography.

## 7.2 Indications in Adults: The Surgeon's View

M.-C. Marti

Defaecography is a dynamic radiological investigation allowing imaging of the anorectum at rest, during voluntary evacuation of the rectum and during retention effort. Several modalities of this technique have been described, but differences are minimal. They concern mainly the choice of bone marks, the way the anorectal angle is measured and the choice of contrast medium.

This special dynamic investigation has provided a large amount of information about various defaecation disorders. Results concern:

1. Parameters quantified as:
   - Central anorectal angle or posterior anorectal angle
   - Anal canal length
   - Position of the anorectal junction
   - Excursion of the anorectal junction

- Anal canal width
- Size of the rectosacral space at the level of S3

These measurements differ according to sex, age and, among women, number of pregnancies.

2. Morphological changes of the rectum and anal canal:
   - Impression of the puborectalis sling
   - Intussusception
   - Rectal prolapse
   - Rectocele
   - Outpocketing and anocele
   - Complete or incomplete rectal emptying
   - Perineal descent
   - Defect in anal canal opening during straining
   - Anal incontinence
   - Persistent anal opening
3. Kinetics of anal defaecation
   - Descent of the anorectal junction during straining
   - Widening of the anorectal angle
   - Relaxation of the puborectalis sling
   - Shortening of anal canal length
   - Posterior translation of the anal canal
   - More or less complete emptying of the rectum
   - Flattening of the rectum
   - Return to normal after straining

Studies of normal subjects and volunteers as performed by Mahieu et al. [33], Shorven et al. [35] and Goie et al. [32] have shown great variability in observed results. Furthermore, there are large interobserver variations in the measurement of anorectal function. Quantified data, morphological changes and kinetic observations should therefore be correlated not only to mean values observed in normal subjects but also, essentially, to clinical symptoms. The data should not be used as the only criteria for treatment. Not every abnormality observed necessarily requires surgery or even treatment. Good radioclinical correlation may be achieved when the patient presents the following anamnestic and clinical symptoms:

- Constipation
- Dyschezia or outlet syndrome
- Intussusception
- Rectal prolapse
- Descending perineum
- Rectocele
- Enterocele
- Anocele and outpocketing
- Incontinence with sphincter rupture
- Non-relaxing puborectalis sling

- Anismus
- Levator syndrome
- Solitary rectal ulcer

One must keep in mind that some of the changes observed may be premonitory signs of clinical disorders, but as yet there are still no data from repeated investigations performed over many years to confirm this fact. One must also keep in mind that *patients* are to be treated, not x-ray films!

Defaecography is a useful technique but not a screening examination. It should be performed only after (a) consideration of precise clinical records, (b) thorough digital examination with the patient in the lithotany position, at rest and during straining and retention efforts, and (c) endoscopy. In the presence of constipation, transit should be timed. Manometry and even EMG may be useful in the event of an outlet syndrome or incontinence.

For several years, defaecography was performed routinely in our department; however, its indications are now restricted [34]. From a surgical point of view, defaecography is useful:

1. To confirm a clinical diagnosis of descending perineum, intussusception, prolapse, rectocele, solitary rectal ulcer, anismus or sphincter dyschezia.
2. To investigate complex associated lesions. Examples include a slow transit time with rectocele and intussusception, and incontinence with rectocele. In such cases, defaecography helps in deciding which of the lesions should be treated first, and whether surgery is necessary. It is also of use in deciding whether colonic inertia should be treated before or after correction of an outlet syndrome.
3. To investigate unclear manifestations with normal endoscopy, such as pelvic pain, sensations of rectal mass and incomplete rectal evacuation.
4. To obtain objective data before and after treatment, whether surgical or not, and to assess post-operative results.
5. For objective and scientific evaluation of the efficiency of the treatment. The films can be useful in the event of medicolegal conflict, should the patient not be satisfied with the outcome of surgical treatment.
6. To select a surgical procedure or to assess its extent. For example, defaecography can help one to decide whether rectocele should be treated via an endo-anal approach or whether the lesion is so wide that a posterior colpomyorraphy or even a combined abdominovaginal be performed.

### *7.2.1 Conclusions*

Defaecography may reveal the underlying mechanism causing disorders and provide the physician with objective data. Defaecography should be employed only when it is indicated by both the clinical examination and anamnestic records. Defaecography is not a screening examination.

## 7.3 Indications in Children

J. Hirsig

Defaecography in children is not always easy to perform and certainly demands a great deal of patience. But if the investigator is prepared to invest sufficient time and effort, important information can be obtained even in very small children. The indication must be restricted to children with significant defaecation disorders, however, because of the high irradiation doses.

Especially in chronic constipation, the severity of the symptoms is often difficult to assess. Preliminary measurement of colonic transit time (see Chap. 13) is therefore usually helpful in selecing cases investigation with defaecography.

The technique is basically the same as in adults. We think that the bowel should never be prepared preliminarily. Since most children enjoy watching video tapes, the monitor should be placed in a position allowing the child to witness the examination.

The information we can expect is, as a rule, the same as in adults. Even if poor cooperation does not allow reliable interpretation of the actual defaecation act, the amount of faecal retention and the severity of the colonic and rectal dilation will be a reliable parameter in children with coprostasis.

In the case of a narrow distal segment, Hirschsprung's disease must be excluded with a rectal mucosal biopsy.

An empty, contracted Colon and Rectum in a child with faecal incontinence who displays continuous colonic evacuation implies severe sphincter malfunction. This can often been demonstrated in children investigated for faecal incontinence in connection with high anorectal malformations.

In cases featuring outlet obstruction we frequently find, to our great astonishment, posterior, anterior and even lateral evaginations as an expression of the terminal obstruction at the level of the external anal sphincter. Rectoceles are also found commonly in children with massive coprostasis leading to encopresis, which must be clearly distinguished from faecal incontinence. We think that the outlet obstruction causes encopresis in children with the necessary psychic predisposition.

Defaecography should therefore be considered in the following defaecation disorders in childhood:

1. Faecal incontinence
2. Massive coprostasis (chronic constipation)
3. Encopresis

## References


1. Mahieu P, Pringot J, Bodard P (1984) Defecography I. Description of a new procedure and results in normal patients. Gastrointest Radiol 9:247–251
2. Mahieu P, Pringot J, Bodard P (1984) Defecography II. Contribution to the diagnosis of defecation disorders. Gastrointest Radiol 9:253–261
3. Kuijpers HC, Strijk SP (1984) Diagnosis of disturbances of continence and defecation. Dis Colon Rectum 27:658–662
4. Goei R, Baeten C, Arends JW (1988) The solitary rectal ulcer syndrome: findings on barium enema study and defecography. Radiology 168:303–306
5. Levine DS (1987) "Solitary" rectal ulcer syndrome. Gastroenterology 92:243–253
6. Metcalf Am, Phillips SF, Zinsmeister AR, McCarty RL, Beart RW, Wolff BG (1987) Simplified assessment of segmental colonic transit. Gastroenterology 92:40–47
7. Kuijpers HC (1990) Application of the colorectal laboratory in diagnosis and treatment of functional constipation. Dis Colon Rectum 33:35–39
8. Shorvon PJ, MuHugh S, Diamant NE, Somers S, Stevenson GW (1989) Defecography in normal volunteers: results and implications. Gut 30:1737–1749
9. Goei R, Baeten C (1990) Rectal intussusception and rectal prolapse: Detection and postoperative evaluation with defecography. Radiology 174:124–126
10. Goei R, van Engelshoven J, Schouten H, Baeten C, Stassen C (1989) Anorectal function: defecographic measurement in asymptomatic subjects. Radiology 173:137–141
11. Kuijpers HC, Bleijenberg G (1985) The spastic pelvic floor syndrome. A cause of constipation. Dis Colon Rectum 28:669–672
12. Martelli H, Devroede G, Arhan P, Dugay C (1978) Mechanisms of idiopathic constipation: outlet obstruction. Gastroenterology 75:623
13. Loening-Baucke V (1984) Abnormal rectoanal function in children recovered from chronic constipation and encopresis. Gastroenterology 87:1299–1304
14. Preston DM, Lennard-Jones JE (1985) Anismus in chronic constipation. Dig Dis Sci 30:413–418
15. Read NW, Timms JM, Barfield LJ, Donnelly TC, Bannister JJ (1986) Impairment of defecation in young women with severe constipation. Gastroenterology 90:53–60
16. Jones PN, Lubowski DZ, Swash M, Henry MM (1987) Is paradoxical contraction of puborectalis muscle of functional importance? Dis Colon Rectum 30:667–670
17. Bleijenberg G, Kuijpers HC (1987) Treatment of the spastic pelvic floor syndrome with biofeedback. Dis Colon Rectum 30:108–111
18. Henry MM, Parks AG, Swash M (1982) The pelvic floor musculature in the descending perineum syndrome. Br J Surg 69:470–472
19. Skomorowska E, Hegedüs V, Christiansen J (1988) Evaluation of perineal descent by defaecography. Int J Colorectal Dis 3:191–194
20. Kiff ES, Barnes RPH, Swash M (1984) Evidence of pudendal neuropathy in patients with perineal descent and chronic constipation. Gut 25:1279–1282
21. Snooks SJ, Barnes PRH, Swash M, Henry MM (1985) Damage to the innervation of the pelvic floor musculature in chronic constipation. Gastroenterology 89:977–981
22. Parks AG, Swash M, Urich H (1977) Sphincter denervation in anorectal incontinence and rectal prolapse. Gut 18:656–665
23. Bartolo DCC, Jarratt JA, Read NW (1983) The use of conventional electromyography to assess external sphincter neuropathy in man. J Neurol Neurosurg Psychiatry 46:1115–1118

24. Beersiek F, Parks AG, Swash M (1979) Pathogenesis of anorectal incontinence: a histometric study of the anal sphincter musculature. J Neurol Sci 42:111–127
25. Kiff ES, Swash M (1984) Slowed conduction in the pudendal nerves in idiopathic (neurogenic) faecal incontinence. Br J Surg 71:614–616
26. Neill ME, Parks AG, Swash M (1981) Physiological studies of the anal sphincter musculature in faecal incontinence and rectal prolapse. Br J Surg 68:531–536
27. Matheson DM, Keighley M (1981) Manometric evaluation of rectal prolapse and faecal incontinence. Gut 22:126–129
28. Snooks SJ, Henry MM, Swash M (1985) Anorectal incontinence and rectal prolapse: differential assessment of the innervation to puborectalis and external anal sphincter muscles. Gut 26:470–476
29. Read NW, Abouzekry L (1986) Why do patients with faecal impaction have faecal incontinence. Gut 27:283–287
30. Snooks SJ, Henry MM, Swash M (1985) Anorectal incontinence and rectal prolapse: differential assessment of the innervation to puborectalis and external anal sphincter muscles. Gut 26:470–476
31. Schweiger M, Alexander-Williams J (1977) Solitary ulcer syndrome of the rectum. Its association with occult rectal prolapse. Lancet I:170–171
32. Goie R, van Engelshoven J, Schouten H, Baeten C, Stassen C (1989) Anorectal function: defecography measurements of asymptomatic subjects. Radiology 173:137–141
33. Mahieu P, Pringot J, Bodart P (1984) Defecography: description of a new procedure and results in normal patients Gastrointest Radiol 9:247–251
34. Marti M-C, Mirescu D (1982) Utilité du défécogramme en proctologie. Ann Gastroenterol Hepatol (Paris) 18:379–394
35. Shorven PJ, McHugh S, Diamant NE, Somers S, Stevenson GW (1989) Defecography in normal volunteers: results and implications. Gut 30:1737–1749

# 8 The Value of Defaecography for Treatment Decisions

## 8.1 Correlation of Symptoms and Defaecographic Results: Consequences for Treatment

D. Geile and R. Stahl

In the early 1980s it was noticed by practising proctologists that a high percentage of patients present themselves because of symptoms mentioned in the literature as typical for pelvic floor dysfunctions and forms of internal prolapse [7, 19, 21], examples being dysfunction in respect of evacuation, forced straining, prolonged evacuation, and a feeling of incomplete evacuation. The sensation of a lodging residual bolus and of pressure that may extend to dull pain in the area of the pelvic floor and the lower abdomen is typical, and frequently regular use is made of laxatives and evacuation aids such as enemas or suppositories or manual aid.

Apart from these symptoms, however, a completely unspecific objective complex of signs is found in a very high percentage of patients. As well as transanal bleeding, which is a typical feature, these signs include mucus discharge, signs of incontinence, perianal reactive changes of the skin and visible changes in the form of the pelvic floor and of the anal canal that range to complete rectal prolapse (Table 8.1). Furthermore, endoscopic examination often shows findings which suggest a dysfunction or mechanical morphological change, such as visible intussusception, complete rectal pro-

**Table 8.1.** Symptoms and signs in patients with pelvic floor dysfunction

| | |
|---|---|
| Outlet obstruction | Incontinence |
| Anal blockage | Soiling |
| Tenesmus | Pruritus! |
| Feeling of incomplete evacuation | Incontinence |
| Prolonged evacuation | |
| Perineal pain | Abdominal pain |
| Constipation | Frequent stools |
| Use of laxatives | Manual aid |
| Bleeding | Mucus discharge |

**Table 8.2.** Diagnostic methods in proctological practice

| | |
|---|---|
| 1. Proctological examination: | anamnesis |
| | inspection |
| | digital examination |
| | proctoscopy |
| | rectoscopy |
| 2. Examination in the squatting position and during forced straining | |
| 3. Defaecography | |
| 4. Sphincter EMG | |

lapse, inflammatory changes of the rectal mucosa characteristic for solitary rectal ulcer syndrome, or displacement of the anal canal or of parts of it.

Of interest is a statistical evaluation of the 1737 women who attended our practice in 1984 and 1985. We found that 634 (36.6%) were suffering from changes or disorders related to pelvic floor dysfunction [8]. This in fact exceeded the frequency for haemorrhoidal complaints (34.9%) [11], so that at least in females and for the time being, the latter (in the past considered the most frequent disorder in proctological practice) move to second position in rank order of frequency. Thus, a smaller analysis regarding only patients presenting in the third quarter of 1985 with complaints in the left lower abdomen similarly indicated the most frequent reason (17/43 patients, 39%) to be changes associated with pelvic floor dysfunction or a descending perineum. These findings led the practice team to investigate the typical symptomatology in 2040 patients in a study limited to 15 months [10]. We found that 779 (38.2%) had the above-described complaints. The proportion of women to men among these 779 patients was 4:1.

As a consequence of these analyses, as of February 1986 and on the basis of relevant literature, we systematically employed defaecography in order to achieve exact diagnoses [1–6, 12, 14, 15, 18–20, 23, 24]. Thus, our examination procedure in this diagnostic field includes defaecography as a routine diagnostic method alongside the five classic elements of proctological examination (Table 8.2; see also Chap. 4) and examination in the squatting position and after forced straining. To complete the picture, it is to be pointed out that colonoscopy or at least x-ray examination of the total colon should precede special diagnostic methods to assess pelvic floor dysfunction (see Chap. 11). In addition, sphincter EMG is indicated in the case of dysfunction of the sphincter or pelvic floor muscles, (see Chap. 14) and is above all of use for the differential diagnosis of muscular incontinence or of constipation of possible neurogenic origin.

Between February 1986 and 31 January 1991, 2079 defaecographic examinations were carried out by R. Hauck for the proctological practice; of these, 1239 examinations performed between 2 February 1986 and 31 December 1989 were evaluated statistically. Again, the proportion of men

**Table 8.3.** Symptoms in patients undergoing defaecography ($n$ = 1239)

| | | |
|---|---|---|
| Bleeding | 758 | 61.2% |
| Pain (abdominal/anal) | 654 | 52.8% |
| Straining | 344 | 27.8% |
| Prolonged evacuation (>5 min) | 342 | 27.6% |
| Constipation | 296 | 23.9% |
| Incomplete evacuation | 275 | 22.2% |
| Use of laxatives | 269 | 21.7% |
| Frequent stools | 149 | 12.0% |
| Occult bleeding | 110 | 8.9% |
| Proctalgia fugax | 72 | 5.8% |

**Table 8.4.** Histological findings in cases of solitary rectal ulcer (SRU) or mucosal prolapse syndrome

1. Non-ulcerative phase: intact surface and fossula epithelium
2. Ulcerative phase (manifest SRU syndrome): flat erosions with a film consisting of mucus, fibrin, granulocytes and desquamated epithelium
3. Obliteration of lamina propria by fibroblasts and non-striated muscle fibres
4. Lamina muscularis mucosae often thickened; lamina propria not or only slightly in flamed or infiltrated
5. Fossula often hyperplastic; goblet cells reduced in number

to women was 1:4 (20.8% vs. 79.2%). The examinations were carried out in a standardised way (see Chap. 5). The symptoms in the patients who underwent defaecography are listed in Table 8.3. It is evident that bleeding and pain were by far the most frequent, considerably exceeding the typical symptoms of pelvic floor dysfunction; the five classic symptoms of the latter showed roughly the same frequency. Objective findings prior to defaecography could be ascertained only in some patients. Among them were typical features of ulceration, of the mechanically caused inflammation that precedes such ulceration, and forms of internal rectal prolapse and anterior rectal wall prolapse postanally (Figs. 8.1–8.4).

It is of note that during 1988, mechanically caused inflammation of the rectum was observed in 78 (27%) of 288 patients undergoing examination for proctitis. Surprisingly, in this case, too, the most frequent source of the clinical picture of rectal inflammation proves to be the mechanically caused lesion of the mucosa seen in solitary rectal ulcer syndrome [9]. Different types of inflammation can be quickly distinguished endoscopically, verification subsequently being obtained histologically. Table 8.4 shows the histological criteria for solitary rectal ulcer or mucosal prolapse syndrome according to Heilmann [17]. The thickening of the lamina propria with the immigration of fibroblasts (above all into the muscularis) is of particular importance (Fig. 8.5).

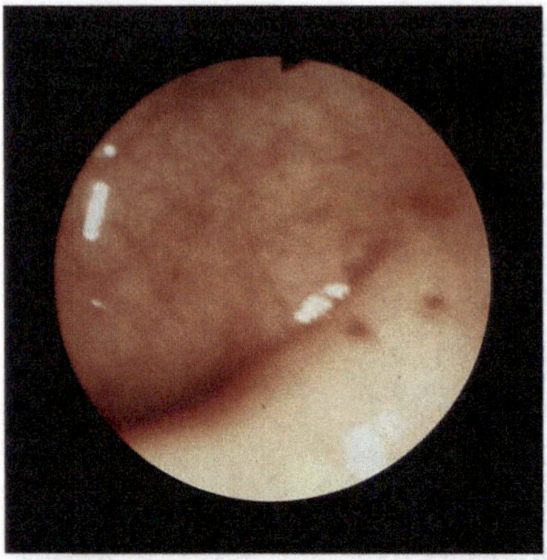
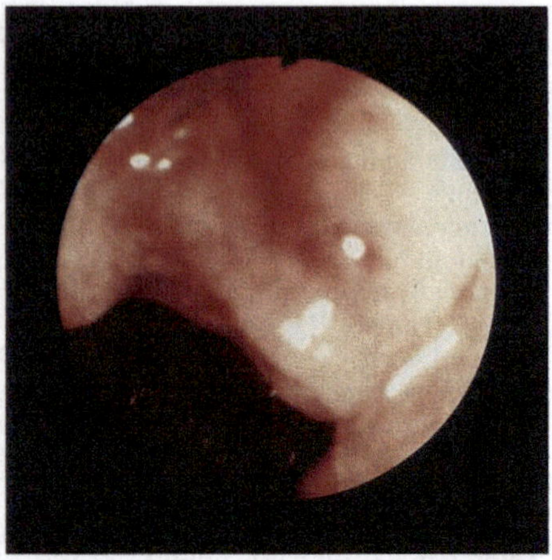
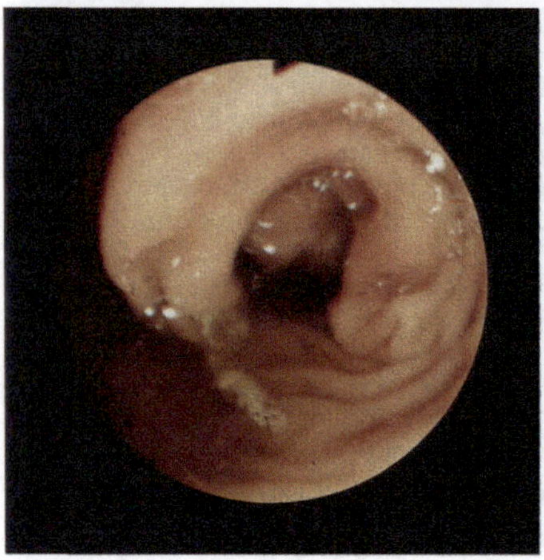
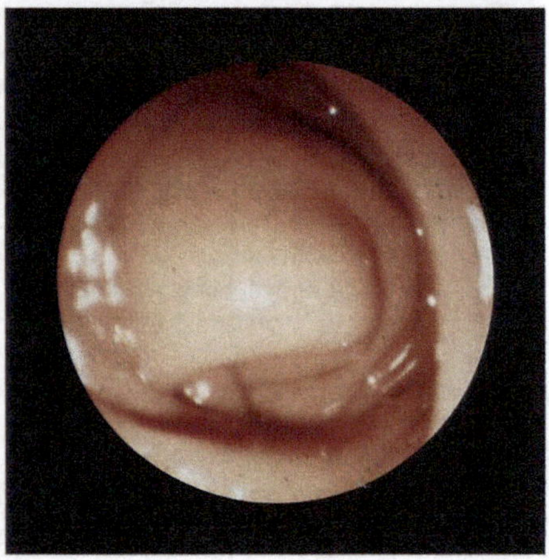

**Fig. 8.1** (*upper left*). Solitary rectal ulcer syndrome

**Fig. 8.2** (*upper right*). Solitary rectal ulcer

**Fig. 8.3** (*lower left*). Circular internal prolapse

**Fig. 8.4** (*lower right*). Funnel-shaped internal prolapse

The defaecographic diagnoses in the entire group of 1239 patients are shown in Table 8.5. The various distinct forms of pseudo-intussusception (displacement of the rectum in the form of z-folding down to the anus, so-called Leporello's syndrome) and intussusception of the rectal wall were observed in more than 80% of patients, followed by rectocele in more than 60% and descending perineum in 47%. The large complex forms of internal hernias which used to be subsumed under the term douglascele and are now called enteroceles, and which present in connection with a sigmoid loop in the rectal intussusception (cul-de-sac), were observed in almost 21% of patients.

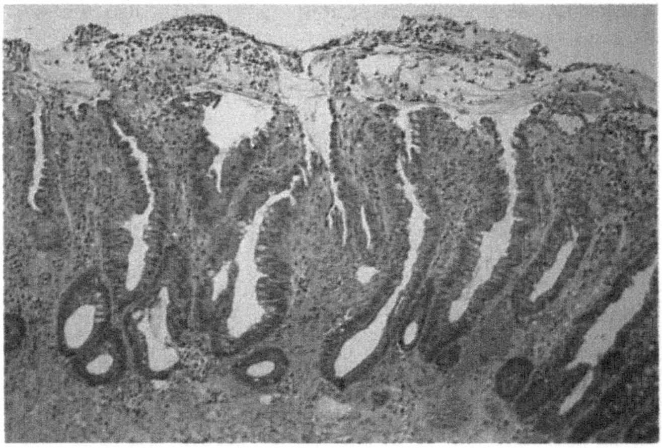

**Fig. 8.5.** Histological pattern of solitary rectal ulcer syndrome

**Table 8.5.** Diagnostic results in defaecography in proctological practice ($n$ = 1239)

| | |
|---|---|
| Rectal intussusception and pseudointussusception | 80.8% |
| Rectocele | 60.9% |
| Descending pelvic floor | 47.0% |
| Enterocele, cul-de-sac | 20.9% |
| Accentuation of puborectalis sling, spastic pelvic floor syndrome | 12.4% |
| Without findings | 3.0% |

This is a surprisingly high percentage, and treatment is primarily operative (according to the kind of change). The spastic dysfunctions (accentuation of the puborectalis sling and spastic pelvic floor syndrome) were much less common. Only 3% of the patients examined showed no defaecographically visible pathological findings.

Recent studies have investigated the extent to which defaecographically visible changes exist in symptom-free "normal persons" [7, 10, 11, 40, 56; see also Chap. 6]. The results of these studies, however, are irrelevant in respect of therapy since *all* patients come to us with symptoms and not voluntarily and since we treat not only the change but also the symptom. Moreover according to our present experience, defaecography *serves to delimit findings indicating operation and to determine the changes quantitatively*.

In the literature we have found only one paper [19] in which an attempt is made to relate defaecographically proven diagnoses to corresponding symptoms. We are interested in this in view of our own work and we have tried to compile such data on the basis of our cases. In an interim

**Table 8.6.** Symptoms associated with defaecographic findings of internal prolapse and pseudo-intussusception ($n$ = 492; 78.2%)[a]

| | | |
|---|---|---|
| Bleeding | 283 | (57.5%) |
| Constipation | 137 | (27.8%) |
| Abuse of laxatives | 126 | (25.6%) |
| Evacuation dysfunction | 125 | (25.4%) |
| Forced straining | 89 | (18.1%) |

[a] Hysterectomy: $n$ = 78.

**Table 8.7.** Symptoms associated with defaecographic findings of rectocele ($n$ = 304; 48.5%)[a]

| | | |
|---|---|---|
| Bleeding | 222 | (73%) |
| Constipation | 123 | (40.5%) |
| Evacuation dysfunction | 104 | (34.2%) |
| Abuse of laxatives | 102 | (33.6%) |
| Forced straining | 67 | (22.0%) |

[a] Hysterectomy: $n$ = 73.

evaluation, 627 defaecographies performed between 6 February 1986 and 3 August 1988 were analysed. The distribution pattern of the diagnoses is the same as that listed in Table 8.5. Tables 8.6–8.9 show the most frequent symptoms for each of the four most common diagnostic results (the spastic changes being disregarded). The analysis reveals:

1. Bleeding is the most frequent symptom in the four standard diagnostic categories.
2. There is no essential difference in the symptom patterns for intussusception, pseudo-intussusception, recto-cele, and enterocele or the cul-de-sac phenomenon – all forms of internal prolapse.
3. Other symptoms occur in the case of the descending perineum or levator dehiscence, though bleeding is again seen in more than 50% (Table 8.8).

These findings give rise to questions that are both interesting and important to proctological practice, and which require practical and scientific clarification:

1. To what extent do the different defaecographic diagnoses in respect of pelvic floor dysfunctions represent varying degrees of one and the same disorder during the course of a long-term illness?
2. Could the dysfunctions of the muscular pelvic floor be distinct from other forms of internal prolapse in terms of pathogenesis, severity and thus therapy?

**Table 8.8.** Symptoms associated with defaecographic findings of descending perineum >3 cm or levator deliscence

| | | |
|---|---|---|
| Bleeding | 224 | (54.4%) |
| Frequent small evacuations | 18 | (4.4%) |
| Abuse of laxatives | 17 | (4.1%) |
| Occult bleeding | 11 | (2.7%) |
| Incontinence | 8 | (1.9%) |

[a] Hysterectomy: $n = 60$.

**Table 8.9.** Symptoms associated with defaecographic findings of enterocele/cul-de-sac phenomenon[a]

| | | |
|---|---|---|
| Bleeding | 84 | (58.3%) |
| Evacuation dysfunction | 47 | (32.6%) |
| Abuse of laxative | 46 | (31.9%) |
| Constipation | 39 | (27.1%) |
| Forced straining | 24 | (16.7%) |

[a] Hysterectomy: $n = 33$.

We consider that the symptom distribution observed by us is similar to that reported in the literature [7, 19, 21]. A further point follows from this: *If it is possible to relate certain defaecographic changes to symptoms and clinical findings, it should also be possible to establish which symptoms and clinical findings may be associated with operative need. It would follow that in patients without these symptoms, conservative therapy should first be employed, avoiding defaecography and the associated radiation exposure. Such limitation of the use of defaecography is especially important in view of the fact that at least 28.5% of the patients who have been examined by defaecography were under 40 years of age, i.e. of child-bearing age.*

We have assumed as a working hypothesis that defaecography will clarify which patients have to be operated on, as well as the kind of operation, and that in the case of the patients to be treated conservatively – that is the majority – only the extent of the pelvic floor dysfunction and the form of prolapse are shown.

We have assumed as a working hypothesis that defaecography will clarify which patients have to be operated on, as well as the kind of operation, and that in the case of the patients to be treated conservatively — that is the majority — only the extent of the pelvic floor dysfunction and the form of prolapse are shown.

In 1990, we examined 445 patients by defaecography (see Table 8.10 for details) [25]. The indications for defaecography were similar to those in the larger patient population (Table 8.11). The objectively ascertained clinical

**Table 8.10.** Details regarding the 445 patients examined by defaecography

| |
|---|
| Age: 20–84 years (av. 49) |
| Sex: 92 males, 353 females (ca. 1:4) |
| *Females* |
| No. of births: 0–7 (av. 2) |
| Hysterectomy: 76 (21.5%) |

**Table 8.11.** Indications for defaecography ($n$ = 445 patients)

| | No. | % |
|---|---|---|
| Bleeding | 233 | 52.4 |
| Straining | 203 | 45.6 |
| Pain (abdominal/perineal) | 149 | 33.5 |
| Prolonged evacuation | 140 | 31.5 |
| Feeling of incomplete evacuation | 94 | 21.1 |
| Use of laxalives | 89 | 20.0 |
| Constipation | 81 | 18.2 |
| Solitary rectal ulcer syndrome | 67 | 15.1 |
| Incontinence | 64 | 14.4 |
| Occult bleeding | 24 | 5.4 |
| Proctalgia fugax | 17 | 3.8 |

**Table 8.12.** Clinical findings in the patients ($n$ = 445) who underwent defaecography

| | No. | % |
|---|---|---|
| Descending perineum syndrome | 210 | 47.2 |
| Intussusception and pseudo-intussusception | 151 | 34 |
| Disturbance of coordination | 55 | 12.4 |
| Anal prolapse | 51 | 11.5 |
| Dehiscence of levator ani muscle | 25 | 5.6 |
| Solitary rectal ulcer syndrome | 8 | 1.8 |
| Rectal prolapse | 5 | 1.1 |

findings are listed in Table 8.12. Table 8.13 shows the defaecographic diagnoses. Unlike in the preliminary examination, a distinction is drawn between rectoceles permitting evacuation and non-evacuating rectoceles since this determines whether conservative or operative treatment is employed. As a point of interest it should be mentioned that of the patients examined by defaecography, a high percentage, i.e. 11.7% (52 patients), suffered from diverticulosis of the sigmoid colon – possibly an indication of pathological mechanisms.

**Table 8.13.** The diagnostic results of defaecography ($n$ = 445 patients)

| | No. | % |
|---|---|---|
| Rectal intussusception and pseudo-intussusception | 295 | 66.3 |
| Descending perineum | 284 | 63.8 |
| Rectocele | 228 | 51.2 |
| Evacuating | 109 | 24.5 |
| Non-evacuating | 119 | 26.7 |
| Dehiscence of levator ani muscle | 112 | 25.2 |
| Accentuation of puborectalis sling, spastic pelvic floor syndrome | 71 | 16 |
| Enterocele, cul-de-sac | 64 | 14.4 |
| Rectal prolapse | 16 | 3.6 |

**Table 8.14.** Defaecographic indications for operation (total no. of patients undergoing defaecography = 445)

| | No. | % |
|---|---|---|
| Non-evacuating rectocele | 119 | 26.7 |
| Dehiscence of m. levator ani | 112 | 25.2 |
| Enterocele | 35 | 7.9 |
| Cul-de-sac | 29 | 6.5 |
| Rectal prolapse | 16 | 3.6 |
| Complete | 5 | |
| Incomplete | 11 | |

The defaecographic indications for operation are shown in Table 8.14, the individual categories being non-evacuating rectocele, levator dehiscene, enterocele or cul-de-sac phenomenon, and partial or complete rectal prolapse. Overall, 220 patients fell into these categories, and about one-third of them had more than one of the operative indications.

We set (a) the symptoms and (b) the clinical findings leading to defaecography (as a further diagnostic step) in relation to the results of the investigation, employing statistical methods (four-field tables, $x^2$ test etc.) to ascertain the level of significance of the relationships. To our surprise some remarkable relationships were identified (Table 8.15). Most of the diagnostic classifications indicating whether surgery is necessary showed a statistically significant relationship to the use of laxatives, which is a typical symptom in patients with the cul-de-sac phenomenon or enterocele as well as in patients with levator dehiscence. Lower abdominal symptoms, by contrast, were typical in patients having a descending perineum to a pathological extent and/or levator dehiscence. Constipation (according to the definition employed by us) was often to be found in the presence of enterocele. The

**Table 8.15.** Relation between symptoms of pelvic floor dysfunction and defaecographic findings ($n = 445$ patients)

| Symptom | Defaecographic finding | | Significance level |
|---|---|---|---|
| Use of laxatives | Cul-de-sac | ($P = 0.076$) | 10% |
| | Dehiscence of m. levator ani | ($P = 0.053$) | 10% |
| | Enterocele | ($P = 0.004$) | 1% |
| Abdominal pain | Dehiscence of m. levator ani | ($P = 0.064$) | 10% |
| | Descending perineum syndrome | ($P = 0.079$) | 10% |
| Incontinence | Rectocele | ($P = 0.049$) | 5% |
| | Descending perineum syndrome[a] | ($P = 0.039$) | 5% |
| | Dehiscence of m. levator ani[a] | ($P = 0.081$) | 10% |
| Constipation | Enterocele | ($P = 0.005$) | 1% |
| Feeling of incomplete evacuation | Accentuation of puborectalis sling, spastic pelvic floor syndrome | ($P = 0.081$) | 10% |
| | Rectocele | ($P = 0.088$) | 10% |
| | Non-evacuating rectocele | ($P = 0.053$) | 5% |
| Proctalgia fugax | Descending perineum syndrome | ($P = 0.060$) | 10% |

[a] Less frequent than rectocele.

feeling of incomplete evacuation, however, was related to spastic dysfunction and rectocele, and in particular to rectoceles *not able to evacuate*. The connection between "proctalgia fugax" and descending perineum is of interest was statistically significant as compared with the total patient population.

Incontinence appeared significantly more often in the total patient population than in those patients suffering from rectocele, descending perineum or levator dehiscence. This is the opposite result of what would have been expected on the basis of the clinical findings. A possible reason for this is that incontinence obviously develops only after a *displacement* of morphological structures.

We then ascertained whether there are symptoms statistically significantly related to the defaecographic findings indicating operation (Table 8.16). It is interesting that of the 11 symptoms that served as indications for defaecography, four showed such a relationship, i.e. *use of laxatives*, *constipation*, *lower abdominal pain*, and the feeling of *incomplete evacuation*. It has to be assumed that the use of laxatives encompasses a complex group of symptoms, so that constipation, evacuation dysfunction and incomplete evacuation are all partly subsumed within the category.

There is no statistical relevance in the symptomatology for incomplete and complete rectal prolapse since in general this is visible using other examination techniques and defaecography is not indicated.

The list of symptoms indicating defaecography shown in Chap. 7 is based on and has been confirmed by statistical evaluation of a larger number of patients.

**Table 8.16.** Relation between symptoms of pelvic floor dysfunction and defaecographic findings indicating operation (total no. of patients = 445)

| Defaecographic finding | Symptom | | Level of significance |
|---|---|---|---|
| Non-evacuating rectocele | Feeling of incomplete evacuation | ($P$ = 0.053) | 5% |
| Dehiscence of m. levator ani | Use of laxatives | ($P$ = 0.053) | 10% |
| | Abdominal pain | ($P$ = 0.064) | 10% |
| Enterocele | Constipation | ($P$ = 0.005) | 1% |
| | Use of laxatives | ($P$ = 0.004) | 1% |
| Cul-de-sac | Use of laxatives | ($P$ = 0.076) | 10% |
| Rectal prolapse (complete/ incomplete) | Visible! (see text) | | |

**Table 8.17.** Relationship between defaecographic and clinical findings (total no. of patients = 445)

| Defaecographic finding | Clinical finding | | Level of significance |
|---|---|---|---|
| Descended/descending perineum | Descending perineum syndrome | ($P$ = 0.014) | 5% |
| Accentuation of puborectalis sling, spastic pelvic floor syndrome | Descending perineum syndrome | ($P$ = 0.020) | 5% |
| Cul-de-sac | Rectal intussusception and pseudo-intussusception | ($P$ = 0.059) | 5% |

It should be noted that the assessment of clinical findings is affected by various elements of uncertainty. In this study one can assume at least that *one* examiner has assessed changes in the pelvic floor and in the rectum always employing the same technique.

We undertook an evaluation of the relationship between (a) the clinical findings that serve as an indication for defaecography (see list in Chap. 7 and Table 8.12; rectocele represents an exception, being dealt with in Chap. 16) and (b) defaecographic findings. Table 8.17 shows the few poor correlations that this analysis revealed:

1. As would be expected, patients with radiologically proven descending perineum syndrome present the clinical findings of such a syndrome significantly more often than does the entire patient population.
2. The descending perineum syndrome is less often present in patients with spastic dysfunctions.
3. A cul-de-sac phenomenon leads to the visualisation of an internal rectal prolapse (owing to the greater mechanical pressure).

The only conclusion which can be drawn from these findings is that defaecography is necessary in patients with rectoscopically visible internal prolapse for the diagnosis of the cul-de-sac phenomenon as an operative indication! In this study we have not considered the anterior anus or prolonged transit time since we have no special experience in this field.

### *8.1.1 Conclusions*

1. After evaluating treatment results [10], we are of the opinion that defaecography is indicated to delimit findings indicating operation.
2. Out of the large group of referring symptoms, only a few serve as a decision aid in respect of the need for defoecography, namely use of laxatives, constipation, lower abdominal pains and the feeling of incomplete evacuation.
3. In all other symptom groups and especially in patients able to bear children, conservative therapy should precede the use of radiological diagnostic techniques. Only in the case of treatment failures should defaecography be performed.
4. The clinical findings offer few indications of probable defaecographic diagnoses with therapeutic consequences. An exception is rectoscopically visible intussusception, in which case defaecography more often reveals a cul-de-sac phenomenon.

## 8.2 The Implications of Defaecographic Findings for Surgical Treatment

M.-C. Marti

We have to treat patients, and not x-rays! Defaecography films should therefore be correlated to clinical history and symptoms (cf. Sect. 8.1). This is even more important if films come from various radiology centers. Furthermore, there is wide interobserver variation (see Chap. 6). Despite a well-codified technique, results may differ due to the choice of a barium paste with differences in viscosity and thickness. Lack of cooperation by patients, e.g. during straining, may also interfere with the results. For example: (a) the size of a rectocele may appear smaller on the films than it feels during digital examination; (b) perineal descent may seem less severe; and (c) imprint due to the puborectalis sling may still be partially present without anismus. For many years I was like St. Thomas, believing only what I saw. Now I do not even believe what I see on x-ray films! The questions that require consideration, therefore, are:

- How far does defaecography help the surgeon in making decisions? (That is: Should the patient be operated on or not?)
- Which surgical procedure should be used?

- What should the extent of surgery be?
- Can the extent of postoperative relief be estimated preoperatively?

Depending on the history and clinical examination, defaecography may be unnecessary or, on the contrary, be useful in deciding between surgical and medical treatment and in selecting the surgical procedure to be employed. It may even be necessary in order to convince the patient of the need for surgery by means of objective evidence, or for psychological reasons to get consequent cooperation in conservative therapy.

### *8.2.1 Prolapse*

A total rectal prolapse is clinically evident and requires surgery in every case. Defaecography is consequently rather unnecessary. A rectal prolapse with diminished anorectal angle at rest, but with good contraction of the puborectalis sling and good anal tone upon digital examination or during manometry, will require an abdominal rectopexy with suture of both limbs of the levator and puborectalis sling during the same session.
A rectal prolapse with a diminished anorectal angle at rest, reduced contraction of the puborectalis sling and diminished tone at rest and during voluntary contraction, will require two-stage surgery. First an abdominal rectopexy should be performed; later on, if the patient is still incontinent and does not respond to muscular exercise or electrotherapy, a postanal repair should be performed.

### *8.2.2 Rectocele*

Evidence of rectocele is achieved by clinical examination. Rectocele may result in constipation with outlet syndrome, or incontinence, but may also be asymptomatic. Furthermore, rectocele may be complicated by more or less severe intussusception and associated with enterocele.
Defaecography may be useful to choose between several surgical treatments. The following radiological and clinical examinations and situations may be observed:

#### *8.2.2.1 Rectocele with Constipation*

With normal anal tone and an anal canal with anterior and posterior walls of equal length, rectocele should be treated by an endoanal approach only.

#### 8.2.2.2 *Rectocele with Incontinence*

Whatever the impression on the puborectalis sling may be, if the walls of the anal canal are of unequal length, the surgical treatment should include lengthening of the anal canal with transverse plication of the upper part of the internal sphincter.
If the rectocele results from obstetric sphincter damage, surgery will consist in a more or less extensive posterior colpomyorrhaphy.
In the presence of rectocele, intussusception is frequently described by the radiologist. It does not require any particular treatment, as it usually disappears after endoanal correction. If intussusception is annular and results in incomplete prolapse, an abdominal approach is necessary.

### *8.2.3 Enterocele*

Enterocele can be easily overlooked during rectal digital examination, but may be proved by simultaneous vaginal and rectal digital examination. Enterocele associated with rectocele can be diagnosed through defaecography. Such situations require extensive surgery, using such procedures as a long posterior colpomyorrhaphy with rectopexy or even a Zacharin procedure.

### *8.2.4 Anocele and Posterior Rectocele*

Anocele and/or posterior rectocele may be indirect signs of an anterior anus in the presence of long-term constipation. Digital examination, CT scan or even NMR is necessary to confirm the diagnosis. Surgical correction with fastening of sphincters to the coccyx, as proposed by Hirsig (see Chap 20), may be necessary in this rare event.
Constipation with a spastic pelvic floor during clinical, radiological and manometric examination requires primarily biofeedback and not surgery. Extensive myotomy and division of the puborectalis muscle should be performed only if every medical treatment remains unsuccessful.

### *8.2.5 Megarectum*

In the case of megarectum, defaecography is useful to prove incomplete evacuation of the rectal contents. If aganglionosis has been excluded by manometry and biopsy, and if sphinceter function is normal, rectal resection may be useful. If aganglionosis is excluded and if anismus is found through manometry and electromyography, biofeedback is an adequate treatment.

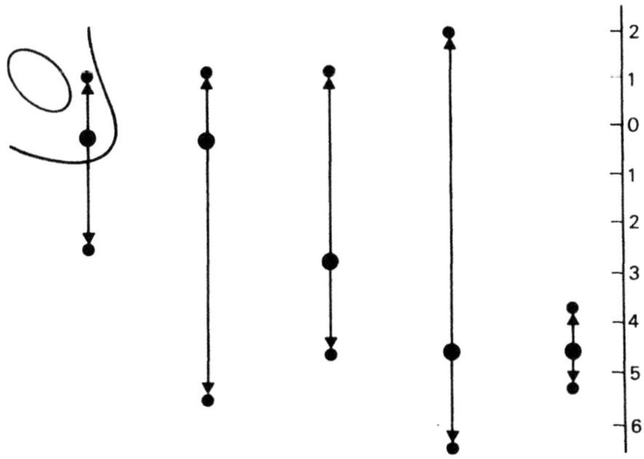


**Fig. 8.6.** Movement amplitude (cm) in normal (*A*) and descending/descended perineum (*B–E*). See text for further explanation

### *8.2.6 Descending Perineum*

There is no treatment for descending perineum as it mainly results from pudendal nerve damage. Its relation to age, gender, incontinence or constipation is not absolutely convincing. Defaecography may help to evaluate the severity of the lesion. A distinction should be drawn between (Fig. 8.6):

A – Normal perineum with a movement amplitude of 3–3.5 cm
B – Descending perineum during straining, but with normal position at rest
C, D – Descended perineum at rest, toned in retention
E – Atonic descended and descending perineum

If the tone of the levator muscles is perceptible, electrotherapy may help. Evidence of a descending or descended perineum may suggest that even after correction of obvious abnormalities, some functional problems may remain unsolved.

In the case of incontinence, defaecography is, in our opinion, of limited value (see Chap. 19).

### *8.2.7 Conclusions*

Defaecography, if performed under strict conditions and with optimal collaboration from the patient, is a useful examination which:

- Provides objective data to explain the lesions to the patient
- Helps in decision-making

- Allows selection of patients requiring surgery
- May indicate the appropriate extent and approach of the surgical procedure

However, defaecography fails to indicate possible postoperative results.

## References


1. Bartolo DCC, Roe AM, Virjee J, Mortensen NJMcC (1985) Evacuation proctography in obstructed defaecation and rectal intussusception. Br J Surg 9:111–116
2. Berretta O, Chaussage S, Coquet M, Couturier D, Bonnin A, Guerre H (1990) Technique simplifiée de défécographie. Presse Med 19:1533–1537
3. Cappellari F, Campobasso P, Scabardi M, Prezalis E, Biscuola G (1983) Valore e limiti della defecografia in etá pediatrica. Radiol Med (Torino) 69:118–122
4. Choi DL, Ekberg O (1988) Functional analysis of anorectal junction: defecography. Fortschr Röntgenstr 149:50–53
5. Ekberg O, Nylander G, Fork FT (1985) Defecography 1. Radiology 155:45–48
6. Felt-Bersma RJF, Luth WJ, Janssen JJWM, Meuwissen SGM (1990) Defecography in patients with anorectal disorders: which findings are clinically relevant? Dis Colon Rectum 33:277–284
7. Fleshman JW, Kodner IJ, Fry RD (1989) Internal intussusception fo the rectum: a changing perspective. Neth J Surg 41–46
8. Geile D, Rath M, Scheidter K (1986) Hämorrhoidenerkrankungen: Grundprinzip der Therapie ist die Drosselung des arteriellen Zustroms. Gyne 7(8):233–238
9. Geile D, Heilmann KL, Rath M (1987) Infektöse Entzündungen im Anorektalbereich – Differentialdiagnose und Therapie. Verdauungskrankheiten 5(6):213–218
10. Geile D, Hauck R, Heilmann KL, Rath M, Ahrends W, Petery K (1988) Differentialdiagnostik und Therapie innerer Pro-lapsformen in der Proktologie. In: Henning H, Otto P (eds) Fortschritte der gastrologische Endoskopie, vol 18. Straube, Erlangen pp 76–84
11. Geile D, Heilmann KL Staber FG, Ahrends W, Petery K, Nirrnheim C (1989) I: Oft als Hämorrhoiden verkannt: Ulcus-recti-simplex-Syndrom. Ärztliche Praxis 79:2698–2699
12. Ginai AZ (1990) Technical report: evacuation proctography (defecography). A new set and method of examination. Netherlands. Clin Radiol 42:214–216
13. Goei R, Baeten C, Janevski B, and Engelhoven J von (1987) The solitary rectal ulcer syndrome: diagnosis with defecography. AJR 149:933–936
14. Goei R, Engelshoven J von, Schouten H, Baeten C, Stassen C (1989) Anorectal function: defecographic measurement in asymptomatic subjects. Radiology 173:137–141
15. Goei R, Kemerink G (1990) Radiation dose in defecography. Radiology 176:137–139
16. Goei R, Baeten C (1990) Rectal intussusception and rectal prolapse: detection and postoperative evaluation with defecography. Radiology 174:121–123
17. Heilmann KL (1986) Differentialdiagnose der entzündlichen Darmerkrankungen. Presentation to the convention of the Bavarian Proctologists' Society, Ingolstadt
18. Helzel MV (1988) Doppelbelichtungs-Defäkographie nach perinealer Sphinkterplastik. Fortschr Röntgenstr 149:629–635

19. Kelly-Mickus G (1989) Defecography – a new technique for the study of disorders of defectation, Canada. Radiography Today, vol 55, No 621
20. Mahieu P, Pringot J, Bodart P (1984) Defecography: I. Description of a new procedure and results in normal patients. Gastrointest Radiol 9:247–251
21. Mahieu P, Pringot J, Bodart P (1984) Defecography: II. Contribution to the diagnosis of defecation disorders. Gastrointest Radiol 9:253–261
22. Mahieu PHG (1990) Défécographie, explorations fonctionnelles. Ann Gastroenterol Hepatol (Paris) 1990, 26:161–165.
23. Sandrone M, Fiore L, Pinna Pintor M, Vaudano G (1989) Possibilitá della radiologia nello studio dei disturbi della defecazione. Minerva Chir 44:1911–1916
24. Shorvon PJ, McHugh S, Diamant NE, Somers S, Stevenson GW (1989) Defecography in normal volunteers: results and implications. Gut 30:1737–1749
25. Theisen J (1992) Wertigheit und Bedeutung der Defäkographie in der Proktologie. Dissertation, Technical University Munich, FRG

# 9 Conventional Radiography, Computed Tomography and Magnetic Resonance Imaging

G. Stuckmann

In contrast to defaecography, conventional radiography, computed tomography (CT) and magnetic resonance imaging (MRI) are not well suited to providing information about functional disorders in patients with defaecation disorders. They are, on the other hand, excellent methods for demonstrating underlying morphological changes such as congenital anorectal anomalies, cloacal anomalies, sacral agenesis and operative complications following rectoplasty. This is particularly true of CT and MRI, conventional radiography being of considerably less value in the evaluation of anorectal abnormalities. The aim of this article is to document and illustrate the value of CT and MRI in visualising both the normal anatomy of the pelvic floor and pathological conditions which may lead to severe functional disorders. The contribution of conventional radiography is also briefly reviewed.

## 9.1 Conventional Examination Methods

Conventional radiographs include plain abdominal films, contrast or double contrast enemas and the measurement of transit time by abdominal films which are taken within a defined time after the oral administration of contrast media (see Chap. 13).

One of the findings most often reported by radiologists on plain abdominal films is "coprostasis". This is in fact a description rather than a diagnosis, and in most cases indicates merely that the patient did not have a chance to visit the toilet before radiography was performed. Only in a minority of cases can marked gaseous distension of the colon, which in addition is filled by huge amounts of stool, be regarded as a pathological finding. The colonic dilatation can be so pronounced that it is not possible to establish the anatomical relations of the dilated intestinal segments (Fig. 9.1).

Wangenstein and Rice [1] were the first authors to propose that when colonic stenosis or occlusion is suspected in a neonate or infant, an inverted plain abdominal film should be used (with the patient in an upside-down position). We prefer a lateral projection with the infant in a prone position because it is a more gentle method for the baby and yields the same findings. In both positions the terminal rectal pouch is the most elevated

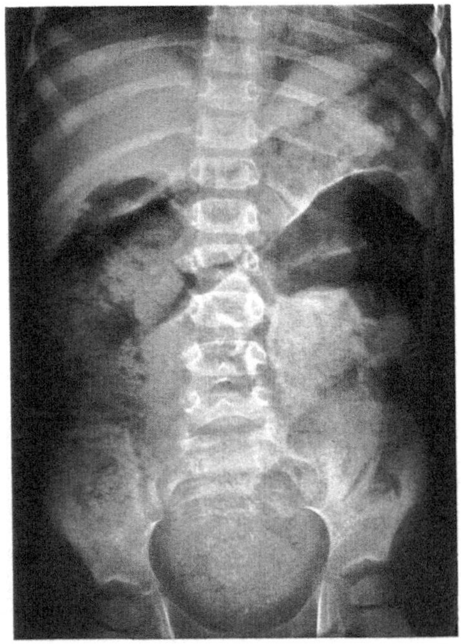

**Fig. 9.1.** Coprostasis in a dilated colon; the dilatation had been induced by neuroleptic drugs

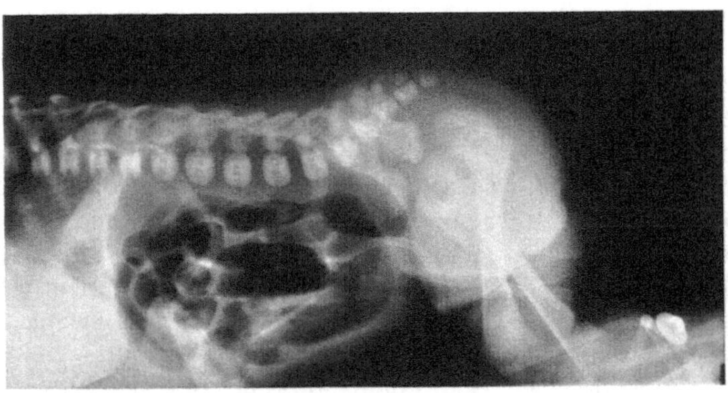

**Fig. 9.2.** Colonic obstruction in a 2-day-old baby. Plain abdominal film taken in prone position and with a horizontal x-ray beam shows no air bubble below the sacrum

part of the colon and is therefore outlined by gas under normal circumstances. In the case of congenital anomalies with colonic occlusion no air bubble will be observed in this part of the rectum (Fig. 9.2). It must be mentioned that this technique is of limited usefulness in patients whose intestines are patent but plugged by meconium, and in whom the ampulla recti itself may be filled with meconium. If in such cases the rectum is not visualised, an organic occlusion of the colon can be simulated. In addi-

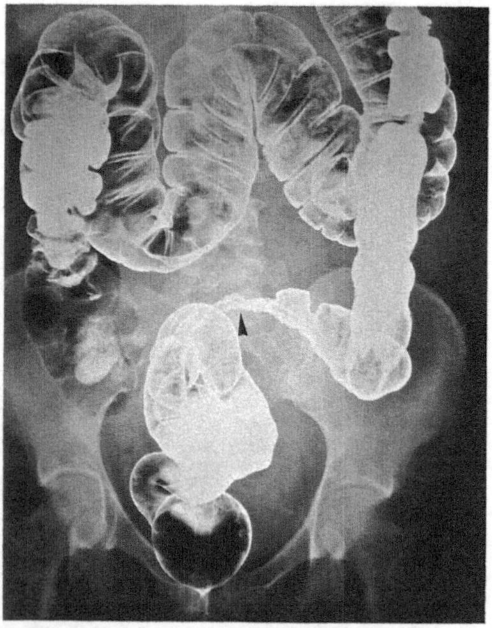

**Fig. 9.3.** Barium enema shows compression of the sigmoid colon by an extring mass (*arrowhead*)

tion, patients with a rectal fistula may show no gas within the ampulla recti although no occlusion is present. One further advantage of the plain abdominal film in the lateral and anteroposterior projections is the visualisation of sacral anomalies which often accompany congenital anorectal malformations [2].

Barium enemas in adults are used to exclude an organic cause of chronic constipation, such as benign strictures of the colon (Fig. 9.3) or colonic cancer. Figure 9.4 shows a patient with acquired aganglionosis of the rectum caused by Chagas' disease. The dilatation of the colon leads to a complete loss of normal haustrations. Patients with neurogenic megacolon (Hirschsprung's disease) are examined by contrast enema. A suspension of barium sulphate in tap water or saline solution is administered to the unprepared bowel. The examination is not to be performed in children who have had deep biopsies of the colonic wall. The typical findings include a small-calibre or normal appearing rectum and terminal sigmoid which lack the myenteric plexus of ganglions, and an abrupt dilatation of the more proximal colon, which is normally innervated. Sometimes the aganglionic segment of the rectum may be very short and is therefore difficult to visualise (Fig. 9.5). The aganglionic, so-called transition zone may widen when preparatory cleaning enemas are administered; the following barium enema is then often inconclusive. A 24-h follow-up radiograph shows the retention of barium and serves as an additional diagnostic sign. In some cases it is not possible to distinguish radiologically between Hirschsprung's disease with aganglionosis of a short segment in the lowest part of the colon

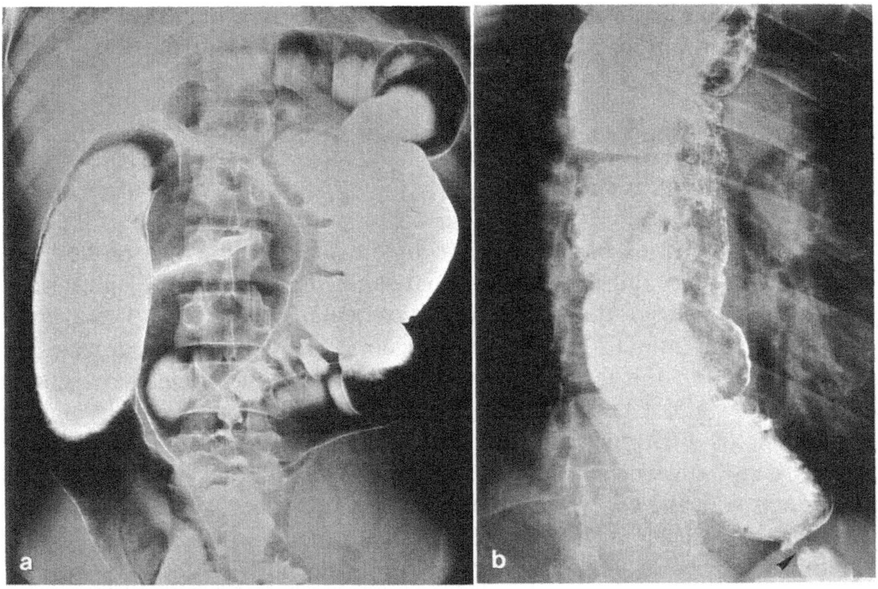


**Fig. 9.4a,b.** Acquired aganglionosis (Chagas' disease). **a** Most of the colon is elongated and dilated. The rectum is narrow and poorly distended. **b** The oesophagogram shows a short stenotic segment (*arrowhead*) in the intra-abdominal part of the oesophagus

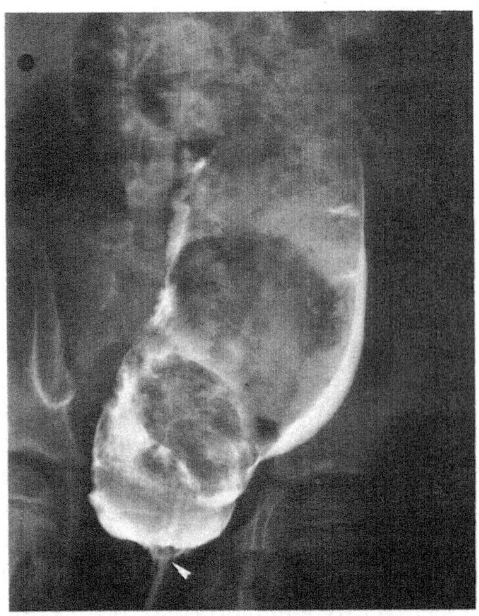

**Fig. 9.5.** Hirschsprung's disease. Very short aganglionic segment (*arrowhead*) and enormous prestenotic dilatation of the rectum

and severe constipation for other reasons. In these patients no transition zone is evident, and rectal biopsy is needed to confirm the diagnosis.

## 9.2 Computed Tomography and Magnetic Resonance Imaging

### *9.2.1 Anatomical Considerations*

The striated muscles of the pelvic floor are divided into two groups: the levator ani group and the external anal sphincter. The levator ani muscle, which extends from the pelvis to the subcutaneous layers of the anus, comprises four muscle groups: the iliococcygeus, the pubococcygeus, the puborectalis and the levator prostatae (in females: the sphincter vaginae) muscles (see also Chap. 2). The inferior part of the puborectalis muscle is continuous with the external anal sphincter, which consists of three layers: deep, superficial and subcutaneous. The external anal sphincter is connected with the coccygeal tip by thin muscle strands which surround the anococcygeal ligament. The anococcygeal ligament, which is a fibrous fat-containing structure, extends from the anus anteriorly to the coccygeal tip posteriorly in a sagittal and slightly caudocranial direction. The two muscle groups of the levator ani and the external anal sphincter form an inverted funnel whose apex is at the skin and the subcutaneous layers of the anus. Because of their oblique course to the pelvic wall, the iliococcygeus and the pubococcygeus muscles cannot be imaged distinctly on the normal axial, sagittal and coronal planes. The lowest part of the muscular funnel, i.e. the puborectalis muscle and external anal sphincter, shows a more sagittal orientation and can be sufficiently visualised on transaxial and sagittal planes. It is, on the other hand, not possible to separate distinctly the inferior parts of the puborectalis muscle and the external anal sphincter. This is easy to understand since even anatomically these two muscles are intimately intertwined and inseparable, forming a functional coherent unit [3].

### *9.2.2 Technique*

Computed tomography is performed in axial planes. The gantry is tilted parallel to the pubococcygeal line, and sections of 4 mm thickness are obtained every 2 mm. The patient is viewed in the supine position after rectal administration of 300 ml diluted meglumine (Telebrix gastro). In addition, a small catheter is placed in the rectal opening in order to identify the rectum. The pelvic floor is imaged from the S5–coccyx transition down to 10 mm below the coccygeal tip, i.e. to the level of the ischial tuberosities. Once the examination has been completed, a sagittal reformation in the midplane is done in order to show the fixation of the external anal sphincter and the levator sling to the coccyx.

Magnetic resonance imaging is performed with a 1.5-T superconducting system. In accordance with the recommendation of Heiken, we use both T1-weighted [spin-echo (SE), repetition time (TR) 260–500 ms, echo time (TE) 12–35 ms] and T2-weighted (SE 1500–3000 ms/90–120 ms) pulse sequences [4]. Transaxial and sagittal images are obtained in all cases. In patients who have an additional malformation of the kidneys or the sacrum, coronal sections are also obtained [5]. The scans are done at 4-mm intervals on the transaxial projection and at 6.5-mm intervals on the sagittal projection. Small infants are studied with a 25-cm (head coil) field of view; other patients are examined with a 40-cm field of view. In female patients a tampon is placed in the vagina.

### *9.2.3 Findings*

On transaxial CT sections the levator sling and the external anal sphincter are well depicted as ring-like structures of soft tissue density surrounding the rectum. At the level of the symphysis pubis it is the puborectalis muscle which is visualised, whereas at a lower level slightly above the ischial tuberosities the external anal sphincter is shown (Fig. 9.6). The puborectalis muscle surrounds that part of the rectum which is immediately adjacent to the prostate and the cervix uteri and has a somewhat triangular shape. The external anal sphincter shows a round or oval shape with the anal canal in its centre. The dorsal extension of these muscles and their fixation on the coccyx are generally well seen. This dorsal extension is sometimes difficult to visualise on sagittal scans because a slightly oblique course of the muscular fixation to the coccyx will simulate lack of adhesion of the muscles to the coccygeal tip. Because of the similar density of the rectal wall and the surrounding muscles, in many cases CT is unable to separate these two structures adequately.

Magnetic resonance imaging has several advantages over CT. First, direct multiplanar scanning by sagittal and coronal imaging is possible. Because of the better visualisation of the perirectal fat, the puborectalis muscle and the external anal sphincter are better seen with MRI than with CT (Fig. 9.7). Vade and co-workers were able to define the mean thickness of the puborectalis sling by MRI for different age groups, from 2.5 mm for 0–2 year olds to 6.25 mm for 15–17 year olds (standard deviation 0.35 mm and 0.50 mm respectively) [6]. This is important since patients with high anorectal anomalies frequently show an underdeveloped puborectal sphincter. If pull-through surgery is performed in these cases, the thinning of the puborectalis muscle may result in ineffective function of this muscle and therefore in rectal incontinence. When failure of a surgical pull-through procedure becomes clinically apparent and MRI shows correct positioning of the rectum within a poorly developed puborectalis sling, striated muscle transplantation may be necessary in order to ensure an adequate voluntary

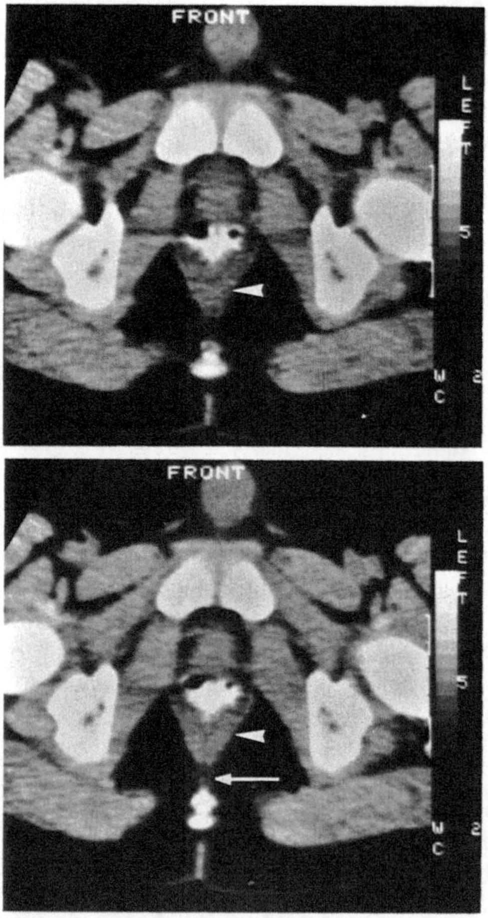


**Fig. 9.6.** Transaxial CT sections of the pelvic floor at the level of the external anal sphincter (*arrowheads*). The *arrow* points to the fat-containing anococcygeal ligament

sphincter function [7]. Another reason for persistent incontinence after pull-through surgery is malpositioning of the anal canal, either eccentrically in the puborectalis sling (Fig. 9.8) or outside the external anal sphincter sling (Fig. 9.9). Both CT and MRI are excellent methods for demonstrating the position of the neorectum in relation to the sphincter muscle complex. The good correlation of the findings on CT and MRI with the findings on surgical inspection and electrical stimulation has been confirmed by several authors [6, 8–10]. Another postoperative anomaly which can be easily identified because of its high signal intensity on MRI is mesenteric fat which inadvertently accompanies the neorectum in the puborectalis sling during the pull-through procedure and later gives rise to defaecation problems by interfering with the normal muscle function [9].

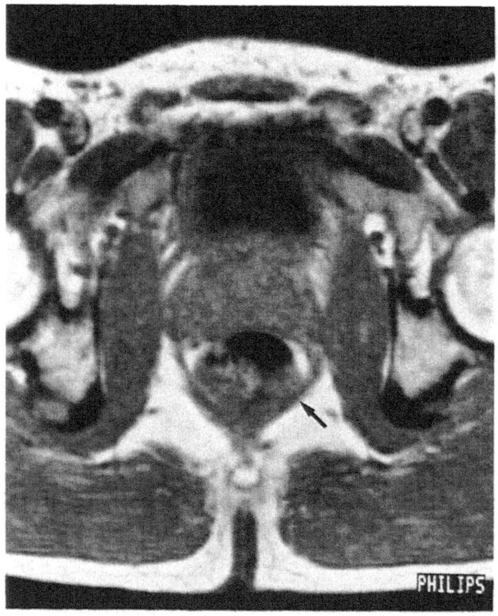


**Fig. 9.7.** MRI of the pelvic floor. TR 600/TE 12. The external anal sphincter is well depicted (*arrow*)

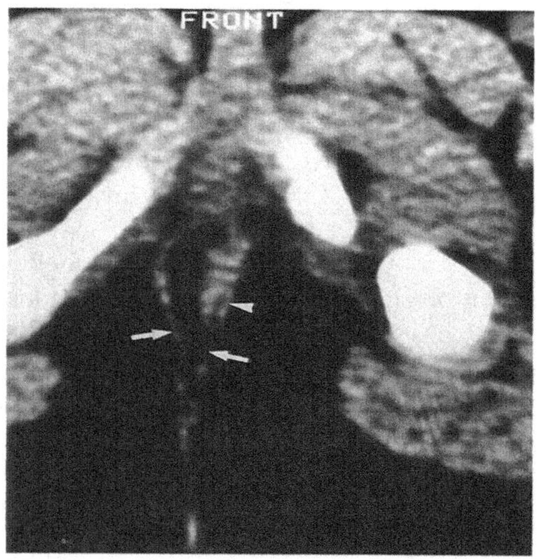


**Fig. 9.8.** Eccentric position of the anal canal (*arrowhead*) in the sling formed by the external anal sphincter (*arrows*)

Sagittal MRI sections distinguish the levator ani complex and the external anal sphincter less distinctly from the rectum than do transaxial sections because of the tapering margins of these muscles in the sagittal scans. A representative midsagittal plane is shown in Fig. 9.10. The dorsal extension of the levator ani and the external anal sphincter is shown as two bands of low signal intensity directed toward the coccyx.

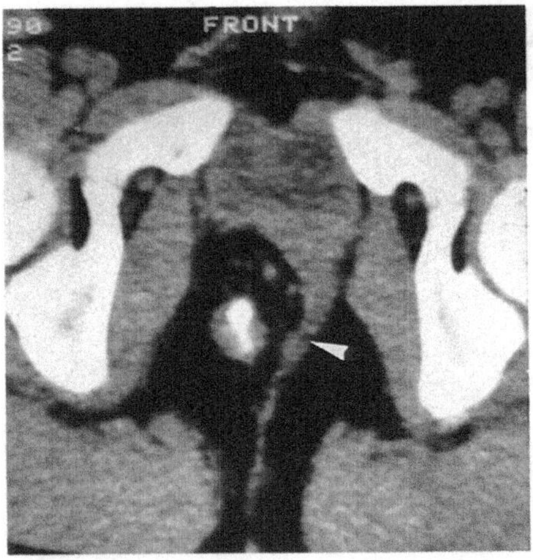


**Fig. 9.9.** Position of the contrast-filled anal canal outside of the sling formed by the external anal sphincter (*arrowhead*)

Sagittal planes are particularly important in the detection of anomalies associated with congenital anorectal malformations. Twenty-five percent of patients with supralevator or translevator defects had additional defects of the genitourinary system or the vertebral column, particularly in the sacrococcygeal region. The encountered spinal anomalies include hypoplasia of the sacrococcygeal segments, intraspinal tumours like neurinomas or lipomas, and the Currarino triad. The latter, which was first described by Currarino et al. in 1981 [2], invariably presents with the symptoms of lifelong constipation, sometimes with recurrent perianal infections and abscesses. Urinary tract problems such as vesico-ureteral reflux, bladder outlet obstruction and neurogenic bladder are frequently encountered. The triad consists of an anorectal malformation, a presacral mass and a sacral bony deformity. The most common anorectal malformation is anal stenosis (Fig. 9.11); an imperforate anus and anal ectopia are also frequently encountered. The most typical sacral deformity is a crescentic defect of the lower sacrum, also called the scimitar sacrum (Fig. 9.12). Other variations are deviation of the coccyx and asymmetrical hypoplasia of different lateral sacral segments. The presacral mass represents different malformation tumours such as anterior meningocele, enteric cyst, teratoma and combinations thereof [11] In 155 CT examinations in chronically constipated patients we found four children with the Currarino triad; one child had intraspinal neurinoma, and another had sacral hypoplasia without an associated tumour. Our patients presenting with the Currarino triad showed presacral masses of mixed density and signal intensity on CT and MRI respectively (Fig. 9.13).

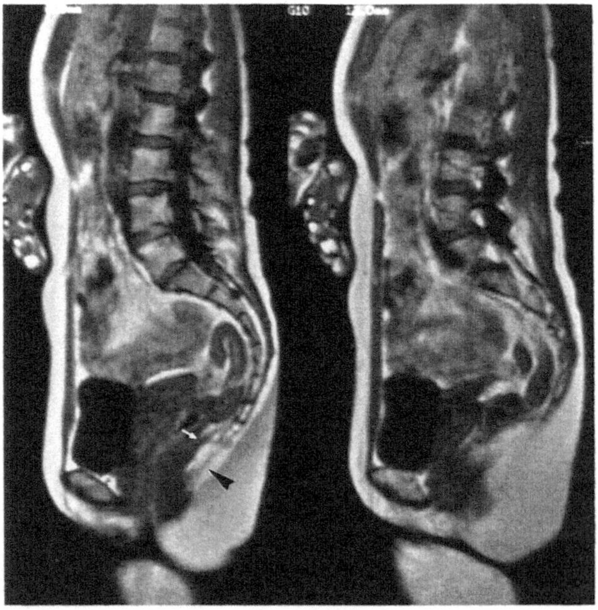

**Fig. 9.10.** MRI: midsagittal plane of the pelvic floor. The dorsal extension of the external anal sphincter (*arrowhead*) and the levator ani (*arrow*) is shown as two bands of low signal intensity directed toward the coccyx

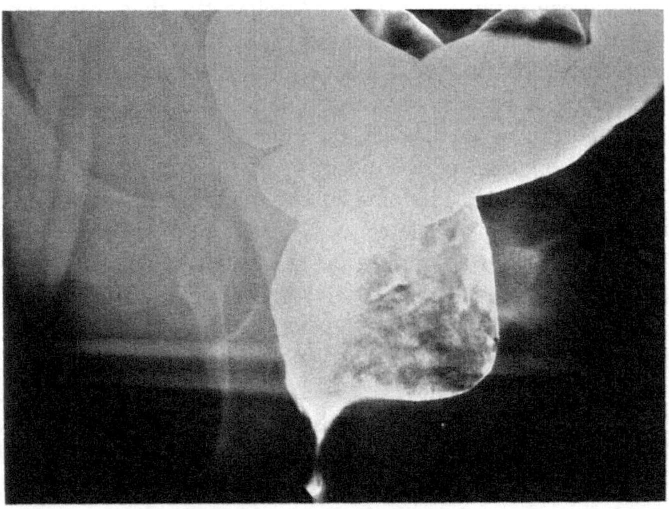

**Fig. 9.11.** Anal stenosis and marked prestenotic dilatation of the rectum in a child with the Currarino triad

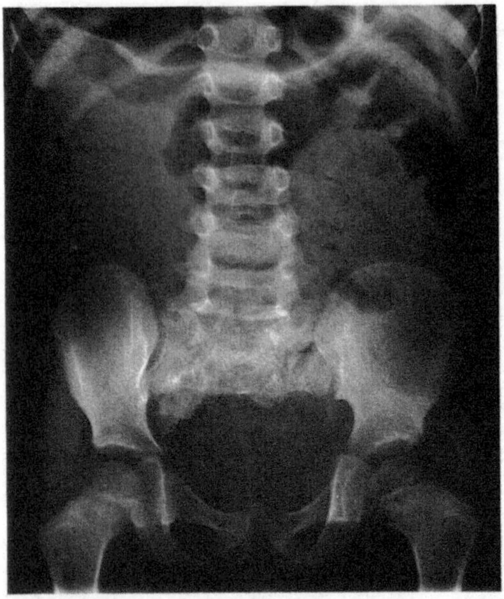

**Fig. 9.12.** Crescentic defect of the sacrum ("scimitar sacrum") typical of the Currarino triad

## 9.3 Conclusions

The clinical utility of CT and MRI in the diagnostic imaging of the pelvic floor has been well documented [4, 8, 12]. Neither CT nor MRI will provide significant information on functional disorders in patients with defaecation problems. However, both examination methods expand our ability to depict the underlying morphological changes non-invasively. This is particularly true for imaging of the position of the anal canal within the levator and sphincter ani muscular ring and of the normal and abnormal anatomy of the muscles of the pelvic floor. Additional pathological conditions like presacral masses and bony anomalies can easily be recognised. In patients who undergo pull-through surgery because of anorectal malformations, correct placement of the anal canal within both the puborectalis sling and the external anal sphincter is necessary for adequate function of the levator and sphincter complex. Comparing the two methods, MRI offers more advantages than CT. MRI gives better soft tissue definition, which is important for differentiation of the puborectalis muscle and the rectal wall. Another advantage of MRI is imaging of the pelvic floor in multiple planes, which helps to demonstrate the relationship of intrapelvic masses to normal adjacent structures. Finally, MRI avoids the ionising radiation of CT in a sensitive area of the body. However, clinically unstable patients who are not able to cooperate or who need metallic devices like tracheostomy tubes or cardiac electrodes not suited to strong magnetic fields have to be examined by CT.

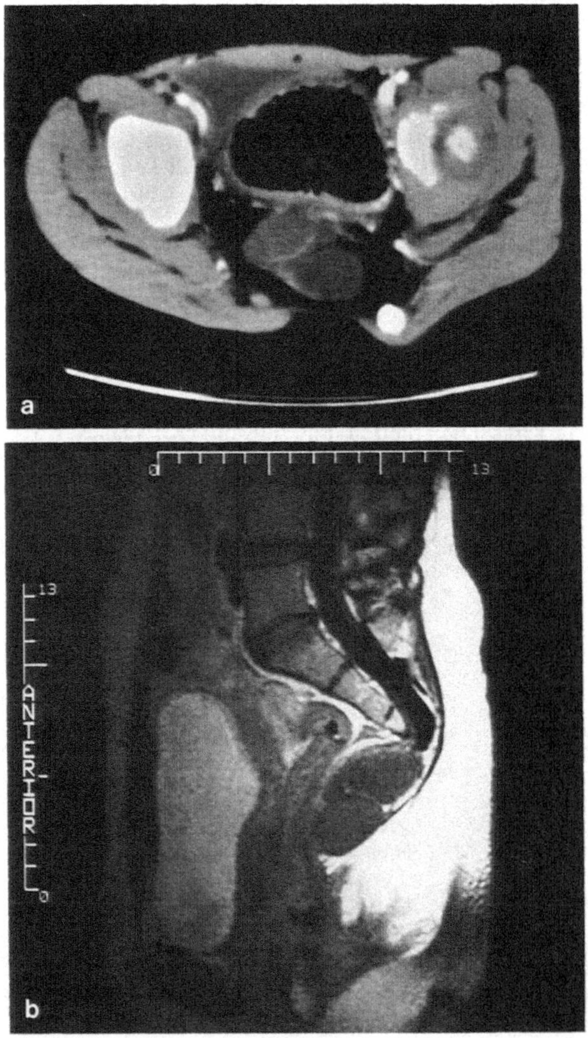


**Fig. 9.13a,b.** The Currarino triad. **a** CT shows sacral dysplasia and masses of mixed density behind the rectum. **b** On MRI (TR 510, TE 16) the presacral masses are of intermediate density. The dysplasia of the sacrum is also well seen

## References

1. Wangensteen OH, Rice CO (1930) Imperforate anus: method of determining surgical approach. Ann Surg 92:77–81
2. Currarino G, Dale C, Votteler T (1981) Triad of anorectal, sacral and presacral anomalies. AJR 137:395–398
3. De Vries PA, Cox KL (1985) Surgery of anorectal anomalies. Surg Clin North Am 65:1139–1169
4. Heiken JP, Lee JKT (1988) MR imaging of the pelvis. Radiology 166:11–16

5. Pomeranz SJ, Altman N, Sheldon JJ (1986) Magnetic resonance of congenital anorectal malformations. Magn Reson Imaging 4:69–72
6. Vade A, Reyes H, Wilbur A, Gyi G, Spigos D (1989) The anorectal sphincter after rectal pull-through surgery for anorectal anomalies: MRI evaluation. Pediatr Radiol 19:179–183
7. Templeton JM, O'Neill JA (1986) Anorectal malformations. In: Welch KJ, Randolph JG, Ravitch MM, O'Neill JA, Rowe MI (eds) Pediatric surgery, 4th edn. Year Book Medical Publisher, Chicago, pp 1021–1035
8. Kohda E, Fujioka M, Ikawa H, Yokoyama J (1985) Congenital anorectal anomaly: CT evaluation. Radiology 157:349–352
9. Sato Y, Pringle KC, Bergman RA, Yuh WT, Smith WL, Soper RT, Franken EA (1988) Congenital anorectal anomalies: MR imaging. Radiology 168: 157–162
10. Mezzacappa PM, Price AP, Haller JO, Kassner EG, Hansbrough F (1987) MR and CT demonstration of levator sling in congenital anorectal anomalies. J Comput Assist Tomogr 11:273–275
11. Kirks DR, Merten DF, Filston HC, Oakes WJ (1984) The Currarino triad: complex of anorectal malformation, sacral bony abnormality, and presacral mass. Pediatr Radiol 14:220–225
12. Butler H, Bryan PJ, Li Puma JP, Cohen AM, El Yousef S, Andriole JG, Lieberman J (1984) Magnetic resonance of the abnormal female pelvis. AJR 143:1259–1272

# 10 Balloon Proctography

M.-C. Marti

Various methods have been developed to image the rectum and the pelvic floor, at rest and during defaecation. Some methods are very complex and useful only for research. To simulate a rectum full of faeces, instead of introducing a contrast medium directly into the rectum, Preston [1] and, subsequently, Lahr [2], have used a specially designed balloon filled with barium. This method is supposed to be more comfortable and less malodorous for the patient and the x-ray staff.

## 10.1 Original Method as Described by Preston

A latex balloon with a wide body has been designed. It has no rigid component, to prevent impalement injury. It is inserted into the rectum and filled with 150 ml barium to simulate a soft stool. The patient is examined in

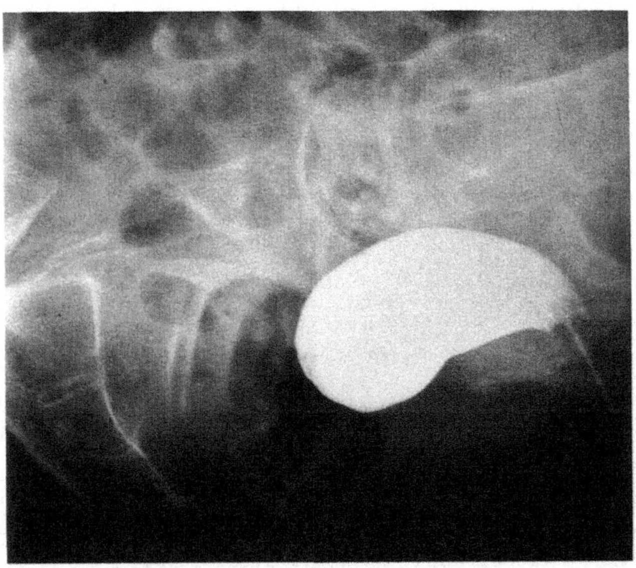

**Fig. 10.1.** Balloon proctography. (From [3])

the sitting position on a radiolucent commode. Lateral pelvic views are taken (Fig. 10.1).
Radio-opaque markers are placed over the pubis and inside the vagina. The patient is then asked to strain and retain while lateral x-rays are taken.

## 10.2 Lahr's Technique

Lahr has developed a special device. He connected his balloon to a bag full of x-ray dye. While moving the bag up or down, pressure measurements may be recorded. The investigator can see whether the balloon is expanded or collapsed at any given pressure. The shape of the anal canal and distal rectum are recorded as well as the strength of the puborectal is and sphincter muscles.

## 10.3 Results

Evacuation of the balloon rather than faeces is more aesthetically acceptable for both patient and staff. According to Preston and Lahr, balloon proctography is well tolerated, quick, clean and involves a relatively low radiation dose.
Balloon proctography allows assessment of: (a) the mean anorectal angle at rest and during straining, (b) the extent of perineal descent and (c) balloon deformity and the patient's ability to expel the balloon. With Lahr's device, it is also possible to measure the anal canal length, the squeeze pressure and the opening pressure of the sphincter muscle.
In 1984, Preston [1] published results after examining 12 patients with faecal incontinence who were subsequently successfully treated surgically by postanal repair, and ten patients suffering from constipation.
In 1988, Lahr [2] published his results gained in more than 280 patients. The data reported concerned 201 cases: 24 of incontinence with prolapse, 87 of incontinence, 26 of prolapse and 64 of constipation.

## 10.4 Conclusion

Balloon proctography has several limitations. The balloon may behave in an unphysiological manner, concealing minor abnormalities. There is no indication as to the overall emptying of the rectum. Furthermore, such mucosal and anatomical lesions as polyps, masses, rectal ulcers, prolapse and rectoceles cannot be detected. Balloon proctography is less informative than defaecography; therefore defaecography alone or defaecography with simultaneous pressure and electrical activity recording is employed instead.

## References

1. Preston DM, Lennard-Jones JE, Thomas BM (1984) The balloon proctogram. Br J Surg 71:29–32
2. Lahr CJ, Cherry DA, Jensen LL, Rothenberger PA (1988) Balloon sphincterography. Dis Colon Rectum 31:347–351
3. Buchmann P (1988) Lehrbuch der Proktologie. Hans Huber, Bern

# 11 Endoscopy and Histological Findings

J.F. Erckenbrecht and A. Rühl

Endoscopic examination is indicated in every patient presenting with symptoms suggesting organic or functional anorectal or colorectal disease. Thus, in these patients endoscopy is the mandatory third-line diagnostic procedure after history taking and clinical examination (see Chap. 4).
If a symptom is caused by a morphological lesion, i.e. an organic disease, a macroscopic diagnosis can usually be made endoscopically, followed by histological confirmation. If proctoscopy yields no pathological findings but the history and clinical examination are suggestive of an organic disease (e.g. transanal bleeding, perineal or lower abdominal pain and mucous discharge), a morphological lesion in the upper parts of the colon must be excluded by complete colonoscopy. If no morphological lesion can be found, the diagnostic work-up should proceed to procedures capable of demonstrating functional disorders, such as manometry, defaecography and transit time measurements (see Chaps. 7, 13, 14).
Typical anorectal disorders are shown in Figs. 11.1 and 11.2. The order of syndromes follows the degree of organic lesion and functional defect represented by a particular syndrome: e.g. proctitis is an organic disease with little functional defect, whereas in solitary rectal ulcer a mucosal lesion can be found macroscopically and histologically, but functional examinations often show an internal intussusception as the underlying functional defect [1]. An internal intussusception usually will not be noted endoscopically.

## 11.1 Proctoscopy/Functional Proctoscopy

Proctoscopy should be performed as the first diagnostic procedure when any of the symptoms suggesting anorectal disease or a defaecation disorder are present.
Proctoscopy is easy to perform and allows the investigation of the lowest 5–10 cm of the anorectum, i.e. the anal canal and the distal portion of the rectal ampulla. A spontaneous bowel movement (an enema should be used if necessary) is all that is needed for preparation. The examination is performed with the patient lying in the left lateral position. A previous digital examination is mandatory. The proctoscopy (length: 10–15 cm) is pushed through the anal canal into the distal end of the rectum with rotatory

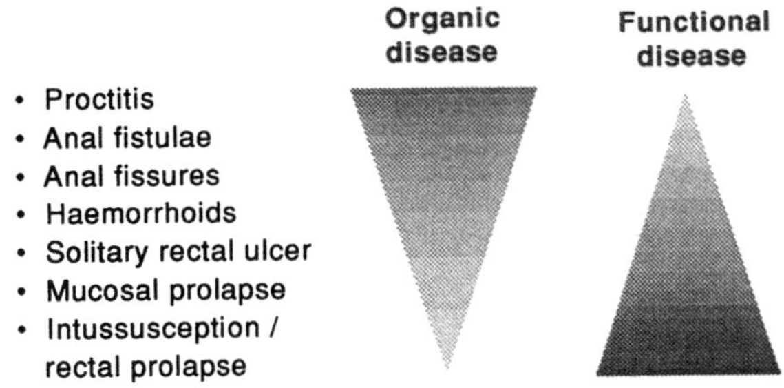


**Fig. 11.1.** Pathological findings in anorectal disorders: organic disease vs functional disease

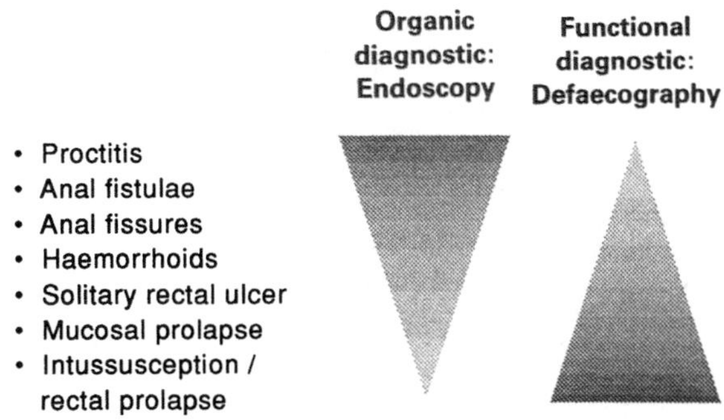


**Fig. 11.2.** Comparative value of endoscopy and defaecography in detecting anorectal disorders

movements while the patient presses slightly. The instrument is then slowly drawn back and the mucosa of the distal rectum and the anal canal, with the rectal venous plexus, is carefully inspected. Manifest functional disorders may be seen if the patient is asked to press during the procedure.

Normally, the length of the anal canal is 3–5 cm. The linea anocutanea should be clearly demarcated and the mucosa of the rectum and anal canal must not protrude into the proctoscope if it is directed to the centre of the rectal lumen and the patient is asked to strain. The rectal wall collapsing into the proctoscope is a normal finding [2–4].

Anterior mucosal prolapse is supposed to be the first sign of a progressive weakness of the rectal wall. The next step is an anterior intussusception, which may be followed by circular intussusception and finally complete rectal prolapse. The solitary rectal ulcer syndrome is associated in most cases with such rectal wall weakness. The diagnosis of the ulcer may be established endoscopically, while defaecography is the best means of assessing the protrusion of the rectal mucosa [1, 5, 6].

Endoscopy of the anorectum does not take more than 5–10 min, bears little inconvenience for the patient and is comparatively inexpensive since the endoscopic equipment is usually readily at hand and has further uses beyond

**Table 11.1.** Pathological findings in proctoscopy

| |
|---|
| Proctitis |
| Anal fistulae |
| Anal fissures |
| Haemorrhoids |
| Solitary rectal ulcer |
| Mucosal prolapse |
| Intussusception/rectal prolapse |

**Table 11.2.** Value of diagnostic procedures for anorectal diseases

| Method | Inconvenience for patients | Expense of procedure | Relevance for treatment decisions |
|---|---|---|---|
| History | (+) | 0 | +++ |
| Clinical examination | (+) | 0 | +++ |
| Proctoscopy | + | ++ | ++ |
| Manometry | ++ | +++ | ++ |
| EMG | +++ | +++ | ++ |
| Endosonography | ++ | +++ | + |
| Defaecography | ++ | ++ | ++ |
| CT/MRI | + | +++ | + |

anorectal disorders. The value of proctoscopy for treatment decisions is high, as most organic anorectal diseases can be diagnosed by this procedure and no further examinations are needed (Tables 11.1, 11.2).

## 11.2 Rectoscopy/Partial Colonoscopy

If alarming symptoms and signs (e.g. rectal bleeding, unexplained weight loss, lower abdominal pain, mucous discharge) are present and are not satisfactorily explained by obvious proctoscopic findings, the next step is to perform a rectoscopy or partial colonoscopy (sigmoidoscopy). Patients should be prepared with an enema.

In rectoscopy, the instrument (length: 20–30 cm) is pushed into the rectum and inspection of the mucosal layer of the rectal wall and the movements of the rectal wall itself takes place while the instrument is drawn back.

The other option is not to perform rectoscopy but rather partial colonoscopy with a flexible sigmoidoscope (length 50–60 cm). The advantage of the latter method lies in the fact that in most patients rectoscopy can only be performed up to 10 or 15 cm, while in partial colonoscopy 50–60 cm will be reached by most investigators [2].

## 11.3 Total Colonoscopy

Total colonoscopy is expensive and time consuming; therefore it cannot be recommended as a screening method in anorectal disorders. Nevertheless, as the frequency of colorectal carcinomas and neoplastic lesions in the right colon is increasing, total colonoscopy has to be performed if symptoms and signs suggestive of organic anorectal disease (especially discharge of blood, be it overt or occult) are present and cannot be fully explained by proctoscopy and rectosigmoidoscopy [7–11]. Further indications for total colonoscopy in anorectal disorders are:

- Age over 45 years
- Lack of benefit from treatment of the anorectal disease
- Relapse of transanal bleeding in spite of therapy
- Polyps found by rectosigmoidoscopy [3]

The patient should be prepared for total colonoscopy by means of an orthograde intestinal lavage with a saline solution.

## 11.4 Histology

During each of the endoscopic procedures, biopsies should be taken from suspicious mucosal areas. Differentiation between inflammation and malignancies and characterisation of the type of inflammation in chronic inflammatory bowel disease should be confirmed histologically.

## 11.5 Barium Enemas

The radiological examination of the anorectum and colon may render information complementary to that supplied by endoscopy. Barium enemas are especially indicated in:

- Diverticulosis of the colon
- Intramural processes
- Impression of the colon by extraluminal structures
- Fistulas

If total colonoscopy is technically not feasible, it is possible to combine partial colonoscopy with a barium enema study to examine the whole colon. The disadvantages of the radiological investigation of the colon are the impossibility of taking biopsies and of conducting local therapy.

## References


1. Levine DS (1987) "Solitary" rectal ulcer syndrome. Gastroenterology 92: 243–253
2. Buchman P (1985) Lehrbuch der Proktologie. Huber, Bern
3. Rothenbühler JM, Harder F (1990) Proktologische Untersuchungstechnik. In: Siewert JR, Harder F, Allgöwer M, Blum AL, Creutzfeldt W, Hollender LF, Peiper HJ (eds) Chirurgische Gastroenterologie, vol 2. Springer, Berlin Heidelberg New York
4. Birkner B (1989) Basisdiagnostik – Anamnese, digitale Untersuchung und funktionelle Proktoskopie. In: Müller-Lissner SA, Akkermans LMA (eds) Chronische Obstipation und Stuhlinkontinenz. Springer, Berlin Heidelberg New York, pp 67–81
5. Schweiger M, Alexander-Williams J (1977) Solitary ulcer syndrome of the rectum. Its association with occult rectal prolapse. Lancet I:170–171
6. Goei R, Baeten C, Arends JW (1988) The solitary rectal ulcer syndrome: findings on barium enema study and defecography. Radiology 168:303–306
7. Ansher AF, Lewis JH, Fleischer DE, Cattau EL Jr, Collen MJ, O'Kieffe DA, Korman LY, Benjamin SB (1989) Hyperplastic colonic polyps as a marker for adenomatous colonic polyps. Am J Gastroenterol 84:113
8. Grahremani GG, Dowlatshashi K (1989) Colorectal carcinomas. Diagnostic implication of their changing frequency and anatomic distribution. World J Surg 13:321
9. O'Brien MJ, Winawer SJ, Zauber AG, Gottlieb LS, Sternberg SS, Diaz B, Dickersin R, Ewing S, Geller S, Kasimian D, Komorowski R, Szporn A and the National Polyp Study Group (1990) Patient and polyp characteristics associated with high-grade dysplasia in colorectal adenomas. Gastroenterology 98:371
10. Blue MG, Sivak MV Jr, Achkar E, Matzen R, Stahl RR (1991) Hyperplastic polyps seen at sigmoidoscopy are markers for additional adenomas seen at colonoscopy. Gastroenterology 100:564–566
11. Nguyen HN, Walker S, Fritz P, Kreichgauer HP, Baum KD, Bode JC (1991) Lokalisation kolorektaler Polypen und Karzinome in Abhängigkeit von Gröβe und histologischem Befund. Dtsch Med Wochenschr 116:1041–1046

# 12 Scintigraphy

M.A. Kamm

The use of radioisotope instilled into the colon or rectum allows excellent visualisation of the bowel diameter and configuration, and also allows the movement of bowel contents to be visualised and quantitated.

In the colon, radioisotope can be introduced incorporated into a liquid or solid meal. The radioisotope needs to be bound to a non-absorbable substance so that it remains in the bowel lumen; such substances include non-digestable fibre [1], diethylenetriamine penta-acetic acid [2] or a synthetic resin [3]. Alternatively radioisotope can be delivered directly into the colon, either via an antegrade approach using a fine-bore tube which traverses the upper gastrointestinal tract [2, 4], or via a colonoscopically inserted tube [5]. For studies of rectal evacuation, the radioisotope can be instilled directly into the rectum. Radioisotope which is incorporated into an appropriate liquid vehicle will disperse evenly throughout the bowel contents. For rectal studies the radioisotope should be incorporated into a semiformed paste whose consistency resembles that of normal stool.

In colonic studies, the use of radioisotope allows observation of the movement of contents which can be accurately quantified. Radioisotope counts within different colonic regions can be evaluated, and the ability to scan frequently enables an accurate assessment of transport to be made [3], which may be of diagnostic value in patients with severe colonic delay (Fig. 12.1). Studies can be performed which demonstrate the colonic response to a stimulus [2] or transit under natural conditions [3].

The two most commonly used radioisotopes are technetium 99 m and indium 111 [6]. The former has a short half-life of approximately 6 h, is cheap and readily available, and exposes the subject to a very low radiation dose. It is very suitable for short-term studies. The latter is more expensive, has a long half-life of approximately 3 days and involves a higher radiation dose; it is suitable for long-term colonic transit studies.

The type of data analysis applied to radioisotope studies depends on the nature and aim of the study. For colonic transit studies, static images widely separated in time can be obtained, and changes in concentration of radioisotope in different colonic regions quantitated. When a colonic stimulus is applied, or when rectal emptying is being observed, the data can be continuously acquired in a dynamic mode which allows rapid changes to be observed.

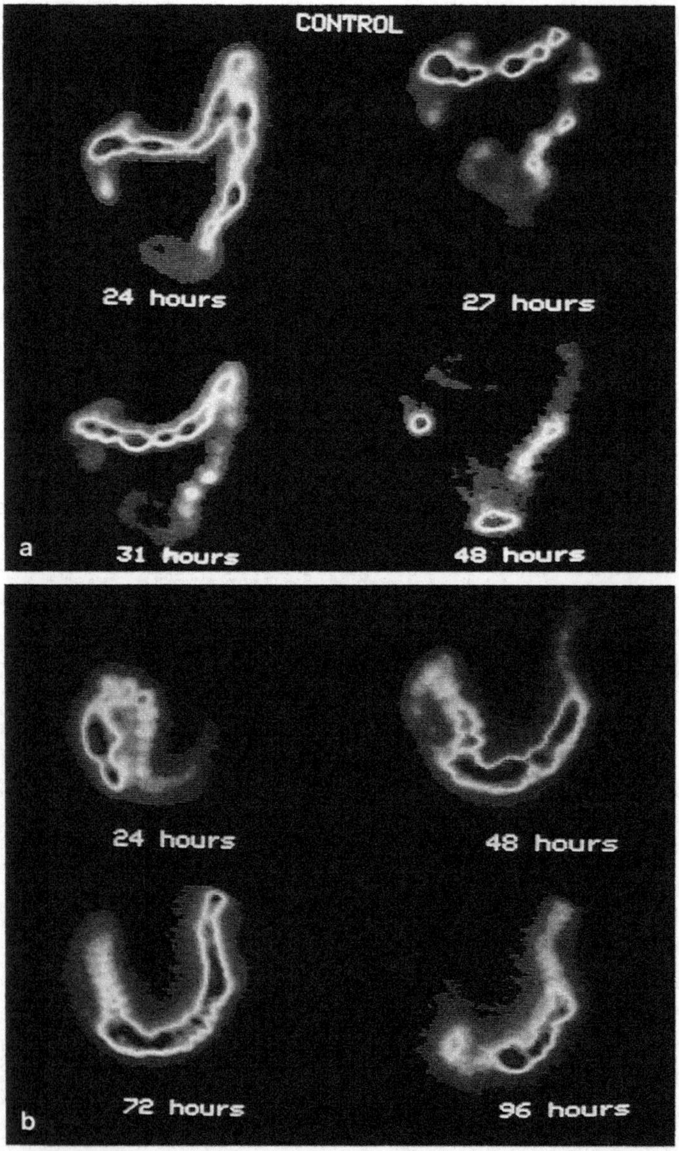


**Fig. 12.1a,b.** Colonic radioisotope scan can be obtained by the ingestion of a labelled meal. In this example, indium 111-labelled resin microspheres were incorporated into a pancake. Sequential anterior scans were then obtained to define the rate of transit of colonic content through different colonic regions. The times underneath each scan refer to the time interval between ingestion of the meal and the time of the scan. **a** Colonic transit study in a normal subject. The radioisotope distributes well throughout the colonic content, so that even anatomical detail such as colonic haustrations is visible. Within 48 h of ingestion much of the radioisotope has been passed from the bowel, and the remainder is in the distal bowel. Movement of radioisotope within the colon can be associated with episodes of defaecation. **b** Legend continues p. 113

When applied to studying rectal evacuation, the use of radioisotope allows the shape of the rectum to be evaluated, although mucosal detail is lost. It is possible to study features such as the anorectal angle [7]. A "region of interest" is created around the rectum which permits quantitation of the proportion and rate of evacuation of rectal contents. In comparison with barium proctography there is less anatomical detail but more information about the proportion of rectal contents which have been emptied. The radiation dose using technetium 99 m is enormously reduced compared with x-ray screening and video recording. The data are stored on magnetic disc or tape. Using radioisotope the patient can be imaged in the lateral position while seated in front of the gamma camera. Radioactive markers can be used to relate bony landmarks to the position of the bowel for anatomical measurements.

When radiation exposure is a major concern and the object is to quantitate the speed and extent of rectal emptying, an alternative to both x-ray proctography and the use of radioisotopes involves the collection of barium or other paste in a tray which is connected to a pressure transducer and chart recorder [8]. This can be performed independent of, or combined with, evacuation proctography. The technique has demonstrated different patterns of rectal evacuation in constipated patients with both normal and prolonged intestinal transit times [8].

A recent application of both x-ray and radioisotope evacuation studies has been the study of patients with an ileoanal reservoir (pelvic "pouch"). The use of radioisotope allows the efficiency of pouch evacuation to be quantitated [9].

In summary, the use of radioisotopes in imaging the large bowel and rectum provides quantitative information for a very low radiation dose, but at the expense of anatomical detail. It may therefore be useful in patients who need to be studied on more than one occasion, such as before and after pelvic surgery, in research studies and in studies of young patients in whom radiation exposure is an important consideration.

◀ **Fig. 12.1** (*continued*). **b** A similar colonic transit study in a young woman with severe idiopathic constipation. Radioisotope reaches the right colon within 24 h of ingestion. However, over the next 4 days it does not progress beyond the the transverse colon [3]. Studies such as this may enable different types of therapy to be formulated depending on the pattern of colonic transit

## References


1. Trotman IF, Price CC (1986) Bloated irritable bowel syndrome defined by dynamic 99mTc bran scan. Lancet i:364–366
2. Kamm MA, Lennard-Jones JE, Thompson DG, Sobnack R, Garvie NW, Granowska M (1988) Dynamic scanning defines a colonic defect in severe idiopathic constipation. Gut 29:1085–1092
3. Van der Sijp JRM, Kamm MA, Nightingale JMD, Walker E, Granowska M, Morris GP, Lennard-Jones JE, Akkermans LMA (1991) Assessment of regional colonic transit in severe idiopathic constipation: superiority of radioisotope compared to radio-opaque markers. Gut 32:A575
4. Krevsky B, Malmud LS, D'Ercole F, Maurer AH, Fisher RS (1986) Colonic transit scintigraphy. Gastroenterology 91:1102–1112
5. Van der Sijp JRM, Kamm MA, Lennard-Jones JE (1991) Simulated defaecation: demonstration of colonic peristalsis with anal relaxation and rectal contraction. Gut 32:A563
6. Kamm MA (1989) Colonic scintigraphy. In: Read NW (ed) Gastrointestinal motility. Which test? Wrightson Biomedical, Petersfield, pp 181–189
7. Barkel DC, Pemberton JH, Phillips SF, Kelly KA, Brown ML (1986) Scintigraphic assessment of the anorectal angle in health and after operation. Surg Forum 37:183–186
8. Kamm MA, Bartram CI, Lennard-Jones JE (1989) Rectodynamics – quantifying rectal evacuation. Int J Colorectal Dis 4:161–163
9. O'Connell PR, Kelly KA, Brown ML (1986) Scintigraphic assessment of neorectal motor function. J Nucl Med 27:400–404

# 13 Transit Time Measurement

J.H.C. Kuijpers

A technique for measuring colonic transit time is a useful tool in the evaluation of patients with complaints of severe constipation. Objective measurement of transit times provides a portion of the information necessary to pursue a logical form of treatment and to monitor outcome. Techniques used to measure colonic transit time can be classified as radiological, colorimetric, particulate, chemical and isotopic (see also Chap. 12). The ideal marker should be inert and non-toxic, remain completely unabsorbed and unmetabolised, be easily measured, have no appreciable bulk and mix well with intestinal contents. The use of radio-opaque markers has the advantage that the passage of the markers can be simply observed by making serial radiographs either of the abdomen or of the stools. The progression time of markers along the colon is an objective indication of colonic transit time. Direct proof that markers are travelling at the same rate as food residues is difficult and has not been obtained for any marker. But the observations that these markers have a similar specific gravity (1.05) to the gut content and that they travel at similar rates to a liquid and finely powdered marker are good indirect evidence [1]. A single value for transit time is obtained if a single solid marker is studied. But, since in constipation the stools tend to be infrequent, it is most convenient to give more markers and to record the passage of a large fraction of them.

The first well-known study on radio-opaque markers was that by Hinton et al. [1]. Twenty markers were administered, and the stools were collected and put in a bag. The disappearance of the markers from the gut or their appearance in the stools was observed by taking serial radiographs of the stools. The times taken to pass the first marker, a proportion of the markers and all the markers were studied. The authors found that the last one or two markers tended to be disproportionately delayed, and that the most satisfactory way of expressing the results was to take the times for the passage of the first marker and of 80% of the markers. The results in 25 normals showed that the first marker was passed by the end of the third day, and that 80% had passed by the end of the fifth day.

A similar technique involves the ingestion of 50 markers and the performance of radiography 5 days later. A total of more than 20 markers (40%) left in the colon is considered pathological [2–4].

These techniques record transit time of the entire gastrointestinal tract, or the oro-anal transit time, 90% of which is considered colonic transit time. However, the approaches that observe the appearance of markers in stools are rather inconvenient; moreover, disease limited to part of the bowel and resulting in delayed local motility cannot be recognised and may even lead to misinterpretation of delayed transit through the entire colon.

In a study by Arhan et al. [5], mean segmental colonic transit time was calculated with a formula which takes into account segmental interdependence. All subjects ingested 20 markers. Plain films of the abdomen were taken every day until the disappearance of markers. The spinal processes and imaginary lines from the fifth lumbar vertebra to the pelvic outlet served as landmarks to recognise the three segments of the colon, i.e. the right colon, the left colon and the rectosigmoid area. Every day the amount of markers in each segment was counted so that the transit of the markers through both the colonic segments and the entire colon could be depicted. Mean transit time was then calculated using a rather difficult formula. Mean transit time through the right colon was 13.8 h, through the left colon 14.1 h and through the rectosigmoid 11.0 h. Using this technique it was possible to distinguish between slow colonic transit (delayed transit through all three segments), hindgut inertia (delayed transit through the left colon and rectosigmoid) and outlet obstruction (delayed transit through the rectosigmoid only).

This technique has not been used widely because of the inconvenience of daily radiography of the abdomen and the exposure to radiation it entails. A more convenient and simple technique reducing the radiation exposure to acceptable levels, the "multiple marker, single-film technique", was reported by Metcalf et al. [6]. Subjects ingested 20 markers on three consecutive days. The configuration of markers was different each day so that they were easily distinguishable. Radiography of the abdomen was then performed on day 4. Thus the progress of markers in the colon was monitored during the first, second and third days, which is most applicable for persons with normal transit. However, if transit were prolonged, a further film on day 7 would be necessary in order to have a monitoring of the fourth, fifth and sixth days. Further extension of the study is possible by performing radiography on the tenth day, the 13th day and so on.

If a person ingests one marker per hour, the total amount of markers in his abdomen increases until he starts to evacuate them. An equilibrium is then reached between intake and excretion and the amount of markers present stands for the transit time in hours. If he only takes one marker per 24 h, the total amount of markers has to be multiplied by 24 in order to calculate transit time in hours. So, if ten markers are administered, the multiplier is 2.4. Our present technique is based on this idea. It is both a modification and a further development of previous techniques. Ten markers are administered daily over 10 days and a radiograph of the abdomen is obtained on the 11th day. The total amount of markers in each segment is counted and multiplied by 2.4 in order to calculate the mean segmental transit time in hours.

The transit of markers through a given segment of the colon reflects not only the intrinsic motility of that segment but also what happens proximally and distally to it. Stagnation in a segment occurs either because a functional obstruction distal to the segment exists, or because the segment itself is atonic and does not contract to propel stool.

Several patterns of marker distribution can be recognised. As mentioned above, besides normal transit through all three segments, there is outlet obstruction, hindgut inertia and slow colonic transit [5, 7]. Between 70% and 80% of patients can be thus classified, but in about 20% an irregular pattern of distribution is inconclusive [8]. An interesting and unexpected finding in several studies was that up to half of the patients complaining of constipation had a normal total colonic transit time, indicating that constipation was not merely related to a low frequency of defaecation [2, 8]. About 75% of these patients appeared to have transit disorders through the rectosigmoid and had defaecographic and electromyographic signs of functional outlet obstruction (spastic pelvic floor syndrome, anismus) [8, 9]. In the same studies all patients with a disordered transit through the rectosigmoid only, had signs of outlet obstruction, which indicated that the abnormal contraction of the pelvic floor muscle during defaecation straining indeed represented a functional disorder of evacuation. These results indicate that there is a role for determination of mean segmental transit time in the evaluation of constipated patients [10].

The quantitative methods in which radio-opaque markers have been used have proven to be safe, simple, reliable and accurate [2–4, 8–9, 11]. The markers can be obtained commercially or can be prepared. The advantage of prepared markers, other than decreased expense, is that multiple distinguishable shapes can be fashioned, which allows one to gauge factors such as the variability in day to day transit and patient compliance [6, 12]. All contrast material from previous studies should be cleared from the colon prior to the onset of the test. Patients should be instructed to consume their usual diet, containing at least 0.2 g crude fibre/kg daily, to continue their usual activities and to avoid the use of laxatives, enemas or other medications known to affect gastrointestinal motility. Radiation exposure should be restricted to acceptable levels. Patients should be asked whether their stool pattern and frequency during the study period were representative of their usual habits. If not, the study may be repeated.

**References**


1. Hinton JM, Lennard-Jones JE, Yong AC (1969) A new method for studying gut transit times using radio-opaque markers. Gut 10:842–847
2. Turnbull GK, Bartram CI, Lennard-Jones JE (1988) Radiologic studies of rectal evacuation in adults with idiopathic constipation. Dis Colon Rectum 31:190–197

3. Dolk A, Broden D, Holmstrom B, Johansson C, Nilsson BY (1990) Slow transit of the colon associated with severe constipation after the Ripstein operation. Dis Colon Rectum 33:786–790
4. Keighley MR, Shouler PJ (1984) Abnormalities of colonic function in patients with rectal prolapse and fecal incontinence. Br J Surg 71:892–895
5. Arhan P, Devroede G, Jehannin B (1981) Segmental colonic transit time. Dis Colon Rectum 24:625–629
6. Metcalf AM, Phillips SF, Zinsheimer AR, MacCarty RL, Beart RW, Wolff BG (1987) Simplified assessment of segmental colonic transit. Gastroenterology 92:40–47
7. Martelli H, Devroede G, Arhan P, Duguay C, Dornic C, Faverdin C (1978) Some parameters of large bowel motility in normal man. Gastroenterology 75:612–618
8. Kuijpers JHC (1990) Application of the colorectal laboratory in the diagnosis and treatment of functional constipation. Dis Colon Rectum 33:35–39
9. Kuijpers JHC, Bleijenberg G, DeMorree H (1986) The spastic pelvic floor syndrome; colonic outlet obstruction caused by pelvic floor disorder. Int J Colorectal Dis 1:44–48
10. Kuijpers JHC, Bleijenberg G (1990) Assessment and treatment of obstructed defecation. Ann Med 22:405–411
11. Ducrotte Ph, Rodomanska B, Weber J, Guillard JF, Lerebours E, Hecketsweiler P, Galmiche JP, Colin R, Denis P (1986) Colonic transit time of radiopaque markers and rectoanal manometry in patients complaining of constipation. Dis Colon Rectum 29:630–634
12. Cummings JH, Jenkins DJA, Wiggins HS (1976) Measurement of the mean transit time of dietary residue through the human gut. Gut 17:210–218

# 14 Manometry, Electromyography and Other Functional Pelvic Floor Tests

M.A. Kamm

Manometry, electromyography, tests of rectal motor and sensory function and imaging of the pelvic floor muscles are used to provide an integrated perspective on clinical problems of pelvic floor function. Many of the techniques were devised for research purposes to try and elucidate the mechanisms of normal pelvic floor function, as well as the pathophysiology of disease states such as faecal incontinence, constipation, rectal prolapse and anorectal pain. More recently many of these tests have earned an established role in clinical practice, providing clinically important information on which to base treatment strategies. Although the main focus has been on the mechanism of continence and the pathogenesis of anorectal disease, there is also increasing interest in urogynaecological disease such as urinary incontinence and genital prolapse, and in the integration of pelvic floor function [1].

No single test provides all the information required when assessing the distal bowel or sphincter mechanism. Most of the tests described are best performed as part of a comprehensive study, involving not only the colorectal surgeon or gastroenterologist, but also the neurologist and radiologist.

In *faecal incontinence*, the aim is to assess the function of the sphincters and their neural supply. This can be done using manometry, electromyography and nerve stimulation techniques. Imaging, using anal ultrasound, provides information about anatomical defects. The sum total of the information provided allows those patients with a sphincter defect to be selected for surgical repair [2] and gives a guide to prognosis in patients with "neurogenic" incontinence [3, 4].

In patients with *constipation*, anorectal physiology tests are of value in excluding Hirschsprung's disease and may be useful in patients with severe symptoms in tailoring treatment. For example, when considering a colectomy for severe constipation, measurement of anal pressures indicates those patients with a weak sphincter who are at increased risk of incontinence if diarrhoea supervenes. Similarly, patients with poor rectal sensory function may fare worse after a colectomy [5].

## 14.1 Tests of Motor Function

### *14.1.1 Anal Manometry*

Anal manometry provides a measure of the strength and structural integrity of the anal muscles. Measurement of the maximum resting anal pressure provides information about the internal anal sphincter, which contributes about 85% of the resting tone. Measurement of the maximum anal squeeze pressure provides information on the strength of the striated external anal sphincter and puborectalis muscles. Finally, demonstration of the presence of the recto-anal inhibitory reflex confirms that myenteric plexus neurons are present in continuity down to the sphincter, excluding Hirschsprung's disease (Fig. 14.1).

Several systems are available for measuring anal pressures:

1. A closed system water-filled microballoon (3 mm) is connected via a 1-mm non-compliant tubing to a pressure transducer. It is cheap, reliable and can be calibrated before each measurement against a ruler.
2. A system identical to 1, but containing air.

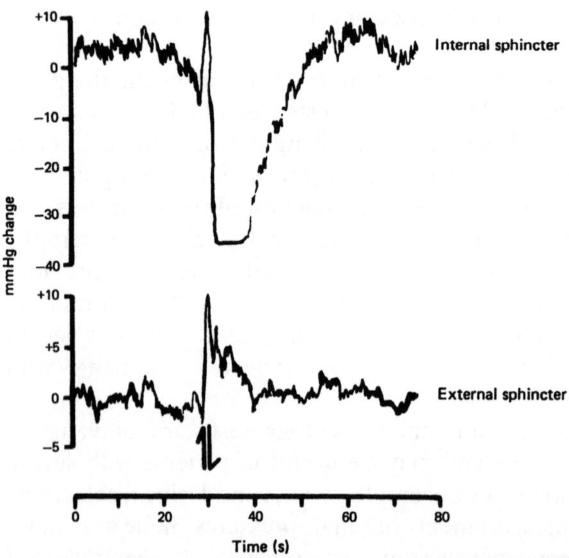


**Fig. 14.1.** Pressure recordings from the anal canal. Distension of the rectum with a balloon causes initial sphincter contraction due to external anal sphincter contraction (*lower trace*). This is followed by a fall in anal canal pressure due to relaxation of the internal anal sphincter (*upper trace*). The internal anal sphincter relaxation is mediated by neurons within the wall of the gut. A pressure probe is placed in the anal canal to record the fall in anal pressure. The reflex is absent in Hirschsprung's disease owing to a deficiency in the nerve plexuses in the distal bowel

3. A water-perfused fine multilumen tube which has six side openings spaced at 5-mm intervals. The perfusion system is connected to six pressure transducers.

In each of these systems the transducers are connected to an amplifier and chart recorder.
Studies of rectal compliance give a measure of muscle tone and irritability. Rectal and colonic motility studies are still of predominantly research interest.

### *14.1.2 Electrophysiological Measurements*

Electrophysiological techniques were originally applied to the pelvic floor to gain a better understanding of disorders such as faecal and urinary stress incontinence. The striated anal sphincter muscles in faecal incontinence had been shown to demonstrate histological changes consistent with denervation and reinnervation, and subsequent electromyographic abnormalities correlated well with these changes. The distal innervation of these muscles, that is the pudendal nerve, is abnormal in many patients with incontinence, and this is thought to result from damage during earlier childbirth. In a small proportion of patients there is delay of nerve conduction at the level of the cauda equina, suggesting more proximal neural damage [6].
Two main electrophysiological techniques, electromyography and nerve conduction studies, are applied to the pelvic floor.

#### *14.1.2.1 Electromyography*

*Quantitative Studies.* Using a single fibre needle which records action potentials from a single motor unit axon (Fig. 14.2), it is possible to determine the extent of re-innervation in the external anal and puborectalis muscles. This provides a measure of the damage sustained by patients with incontinence, and patients with perineal descent who strain excessively during defaecation.

*Pattern of Muscle Behaviour.* Using a concentric EMG needle which samples the activity of many motor units simultaneously, it is possible to record whether the pelvic floor muscles are relaxing or contracting during defaecation or straining. This has demonstrated that many patients with constipation, and some with rectal prolapse and solitary ulcer syndrome, contract their striated pelvic floor muscles inappropriately, rather than relax them [7] (Fig. 14.3). Although this was previously believed to be part of the primary defaecation disorder, it is now recognised that it may be a secondary disorder which results from rectal–anal incoordination (see Chap. 1).

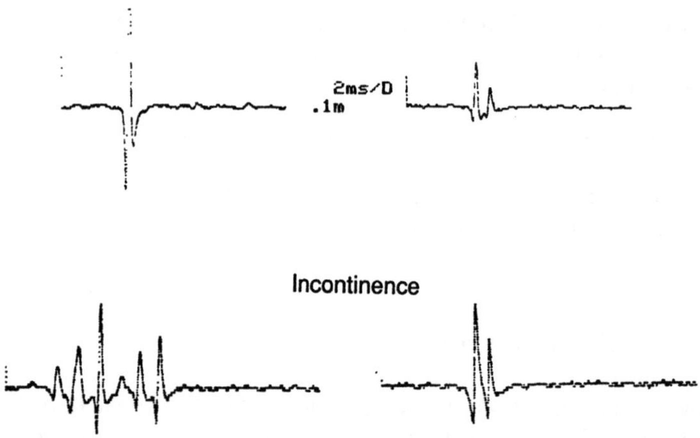


**Fig. 14.2.** Recording of action potentials from a single motor unit in the external anal sphincter from a healthy normal subject (*above*) and a patient with neurogenic faecal incontinence (*below*). A single neuron normally innervates few muscle fibres, but as denervation and reinnervation occur, each neuron supplies a greater number of muscle fibres which contract at slightly different times, resulting in a broader action potential of longer duration which contains more peaks

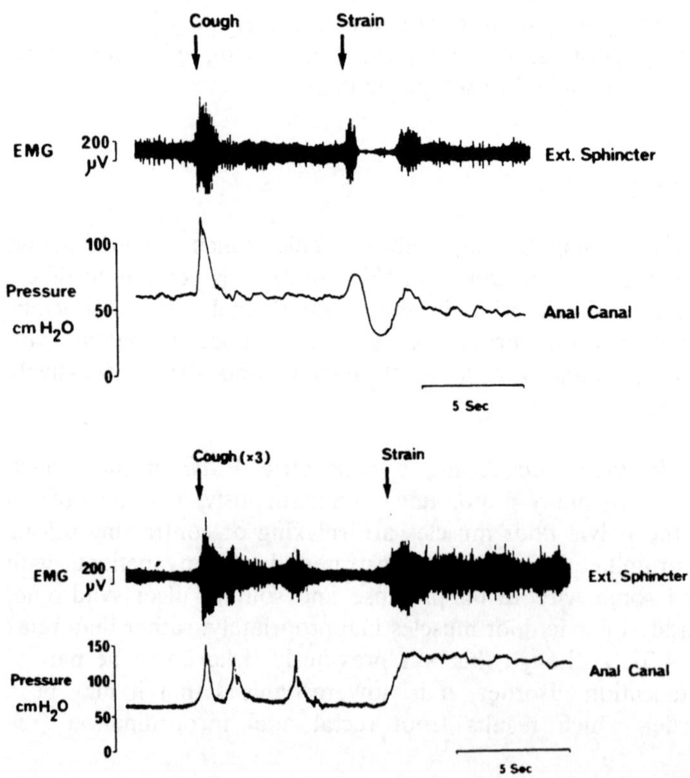

Some young women with urinary retention appear to have a disturbance of urinary sphincter relaxation [8]. Electromyography of the striated urethral sphincter muscle demonstrates characteristic decelerating bursts of muscle activity. These women may have associated polycystic ovaries, and the disturbance of the urinary sphincter electrical activity is postulated to relate to an altered local concentration of progesterone.

*Presence of Muscle Defects.* Concentric needle electromyography can be used to map the external anal sphincter. This provides direct evidence for the presence of a defect in the sphincter which may follow childbirth, surgical or other trauma. Accurate mapping provides valuable information which allows a sphincter repair to be undertaken. Mapping can also determine the presence and location of the external sphincter in patients with an imperforate anus, many cases of which have been previously repaired in childhood. Often the bowel has been brought out in the incorrect position, rather than through the striated sphincter, and relocation of the bowel may improve continence. Recently anal endosonography has also been used to map the sphincter and demonstrate defects; the results correlate closely with those of electromyography.

### *14.1.2.2 Nerve Conduction Studies*

*Distal Pudendal Nerve Conduction.* The electromyographic abnormalities in the pelvic floor muscles result from a disturbance in their nerve supply. The pudendal nerve can be stimulated transrectally as it lies on the ischial spine, using a finger-mounted stimulating bipolar electrode [9, 10] (Fig. 14.4). The resulting contraction can be recorded in the external anal sphincter using a further set of electrodes, and the nerve latency time measured. In patients with faecal incontinence this nerve latency is increased. Furthermore, in the case of obstetric sphincter injury, evidence of sphincter denervation (prolonged pudendal latency) is of direct prognostic importance since surgical repair in the presence of marked denervation is usually less successful [3, 4]. The innervation of the periurethral striated muscle can also be evaluated using the same stimulating electrodes and recording the latency using a bipolar electrode placed in the urethra. This perineal nerve latency is prolonged in patients with stress urinary incontinence [11].

◀ **Fig. 14.3.** The striated muscles of the pelvic floor normally relax during defaecation straining (*upper trace*). This correlates with inhibition of striated muscle activity, which can be recorded electrically and is accompanied by a fall in anal pressure due to inhibition of both smooth and striated muscle activity. Patients with severe constipation (*lower trace*) often paradoxically contract the striated pelvic floor muscles, causing an increase in anal canal pressure. This may not be of primary importance in causing the constipation, however. (Preston and Lennard-Jones [7])

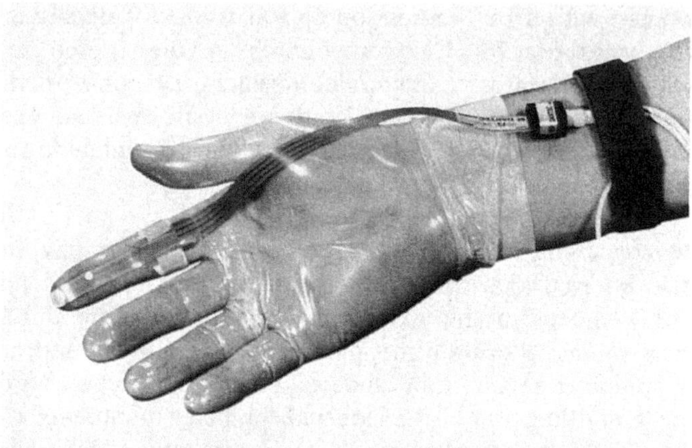

**Fig. 14.4.** Stimulation of the pudendal nerve per-rectally is possible using a bipolar electrode situated on the end of a finger glove. A further two electrodes record the contraction of the superficial external anal sphincter. The latency time for this contraction can then be measured. Prolongation of this latency reflects pudendal nerve damage. This information is of prognostic significance when considering surgical treatment for neurogenic faecal incontinence

*Proximal Nerve Conduction.* Stimulation of the motor nerve roots in the spinal canal can be achieved using electrical or magnetic stimulation over the L1 and L4 spinal levels. The time taken for the nerve conduction to the pelvic floor muscles can be measured, enabling proximal lesions in the spinal canal to be recognised [10].

## 14.2 Tests of Sensory Function

Tests of sensory function provide insight into anal and rectal denervation. Patients with idiopathic (neurogenic) faecal incontinence [12], as well as incontinence from other neurological causes such as diabetes mellitus [13] or spinal cord disease, have decreased anal sensory function. Patients with incontinence [14] and constipation [15] have a decreased rectal sensitivity, reflecting visceral neural damage.

Rectal sensation can be assessed using a balloon to measure the response to distension [16]. The stages of sensory discrimination are: initial sensation or sensory threshold, urgency and maximum tolerated volume (or pain). An alternative means of assessing rectal sensation is by the use of a bipolar electrode to measure the electrical sensory threshold [15] (Fig. 14.5).

Anal sensation can be evaluated using the same bipolar electrode, but with different stimulation parameters [12].

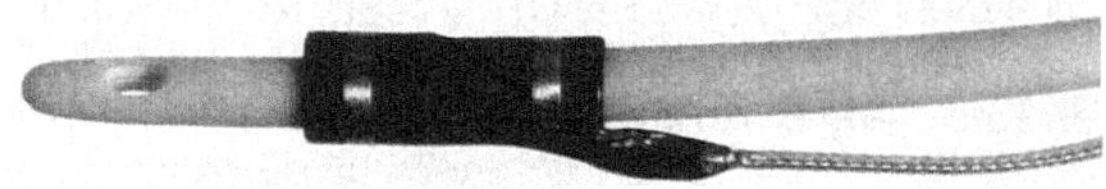

**Fig. 14.5.** A bipolar ring electrode, suitable for recording the perineal nerve terminal motor latencies in the urethra and also for stimulating the rectum or anal canal as a test of mucosal electrosensitivity

## 14.3 Imaging

The new technique of *anal endosonography* enables the sphincter mechanism to be imaged directly for the first time [17] (see also Chap. 2). The internal anal sphincter, the external anal sphincter and scarring in the perisphincteric tissue from previous trauma can all be visualised using this technique. The technique is of value in assessing patients with incontinence [2], fistulae and internal anal sphincter myopathies [18]. Other methods available to image the sphincter complex include CT scanning and MRI scanning (see also Chap. 9).

## References


1. Kamm MA (1990) Constipation, incontinence, and relationship of anterior and posterior pelvic floor pathology. Overlap of urology, gynaecology and coloproctology. Riv Ital Colon Proctol 9:117–120
2. Law PJ, Kamm MA, Bartram CI (1991) Anal endosonography in the investigation of faecal incontinence. Br J Surg 78:312–314
3. Laurberg S, Swash M, Henry MM (1988) Delayed external sphincter repair for obstetric tear. Br J Surg 75:786–788
4. Jacobs PPM, Scheuer M, Kuijpers JHC, Vingerhoets MH (1990) Obstetric faecal incontincence. Role of pelivc floor denervation and results of delayed sphincter repair. Dis Colon Rectum 33:494–497
5. Akervall S, Fasth S, Nordgren S, Oresland T, Hulten L (1988) The functional results after colectomy and ileorectal anastomosis for severe constipation (Arbuthnot Lane's disease) as related to rectal sensory function. Int J Colorectal Dis 3:96–101
6. Henry MM, Swash M (eds) (1985) Coloproctology and the pelvic floor. Butterworths, London
7. Preston DM, Lennard-Jones JE (1985) Anismus in chronic constipation. Dig Dis Sci 30:413–418
8. Fowler CJ, Christmas TJ, Chapple CR, Fitzmaurice Parkhouse H, Kirby RS, Jacobs HS (1988) Abnormal electromyographic activity of the urethral sphincter, voiding dysfunction, and polycystic ovaries: a new syndrome? Br Med J 297:1436
9. Henry MM (1988) Neurophysiological assessment of the pelvic floor. Gut 29:1–4

10. Henry MM, Snooks SJ, Barnes PRH, Swash M (1985) Investigation of disorders of the anorectum and colon. Ann R Coll Surg Engl 67:355–360
11. Snooks SJ, Badenoch DF, Tiptaft RC, Swash M (1985) Perineal nerve damage in genuine stress urinary incontinence. Br J Urol 57:422–426
12. Roe AM, Bartolo DCC, Mortensen NJ (1986) New method for assessment of anal sensation in various anorectal disorders. Br J Surg 73:310–312
13. Rogers J, Levy DM, Henry MM, Misiewicz JJ (1988) Pelvic floor neuropathy: a comparative study of diabetes mellitus and idiopathic faecal incontinence. Gut 29:756–761
14. Speakman CTM, Kamm MA (1991) Abnormal visceral autonomic sensation in neurogenic faecal incontinence. GUT 32:A 574
15. Kamm MA, Lennard-Jones JE (1990) Rectal mucosal electrosensory testing. Evidence for a sensory neuropathy in severe constipation. Dis Colon Rectum 33:419–423
16. Farthing MJG, Lennard-Jones JE (1978) Sensibility of the rectum to distension and the anorectal distension reflex in ulcerative colitis. Gut 19:64–69
17. Law PJ, Bartram CI (1989) Anal endosonography: technique and normal anatomy. Gastrointest Radiol 14:349–353
18. Kamm MA, Hoyle CVH, Burleigh D, Law PJ, Swash M, Martin JE, Nicholls RJ, Northover JMA (1991) Hereditary internal anal sphincter myopathy causing proctalgia fugax and constipation. A newly identified condition. Gastroenterology 100:805–810

# 15 Rectal Prolapse

## 15.1 Rectal Intussusception, Prolapse and Solitary Rectal Ulcer: The Radiologists View

P.H.G. Mahieu

### *15.1.1 Rectal Intussusception and Prolapse*

#### *15.1.1.1 Introduction*

Rectal intussusception is the funnel-shaped infolding of the rectum during straining to defaecate. Rectal intussusception has also been called internal intussusception, internal prolapse of the rectum and occult rectal prolapse. The worsening of this functional disorder may lead to full-thickness external rectal prolapse, also called overt prolapse, which is the exteriorisation of the rectal intussusceptum through the anal canal.
Defaecography attempts to mimic the natural expulsion of faeces from the rectum [1]. It is now recognised as the method of choice for diagnosing functional disorders of rectal evacuation such as intussusception, sometimes associated with rectocele, descent of the perineum and incontinence or dyskinaesia of the pelvic muscles, especially hypertony or non-relaxation of the puborectalis muscle.
The most frequently reported symptoms in cases of rectal intussusception or prolapse are rectal pressure (tenesmus), straining, terminal constipation, pelvic pain, mucous and blood discharge, incomplete evacuation, necessity of digital manoeuvres to achieve rectal emptying and incontinence.
It is interesting to note that rectal intussusception has been found on defaecography in normal subjects [2], so that it requires a long-term follow-up to determine its significance and to define the proper treatment.

#### *15.1.1.2 Radiological Findings at Defaecography*

*Full-Thickness Rectal Intussusception and Prolapse*. According to Broden and Snellman [3], complete rectal prolapse only constitutes the end-point,

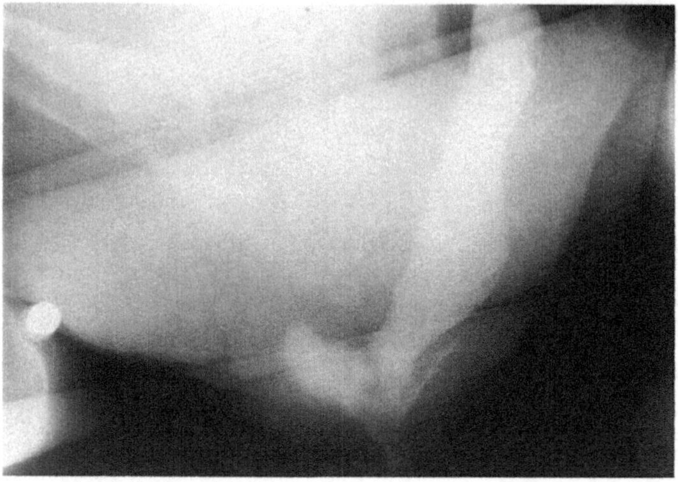

**Fig. 15.1.** Full-thickness proximal intrarectal intussusception. The starting point of the infolding of the rectal wall is located 6–8 cm from the anal verge and the fold is more than 5 mm thick. (Read images from *left to right*)

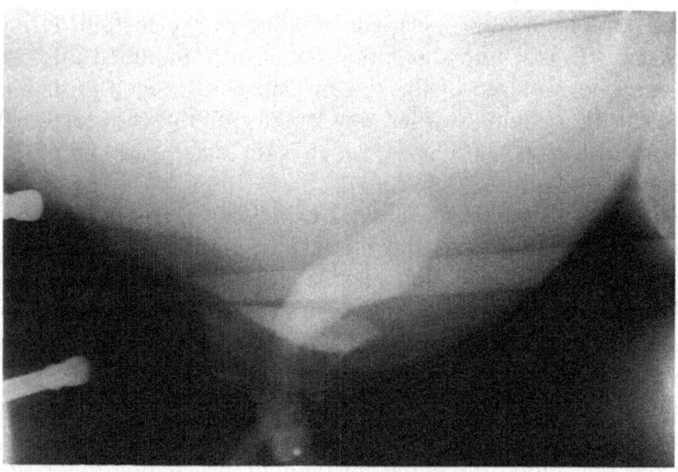

**Fig. 15.2.** Full-thickness intra-anal rectal intussusception. The apex of the infolding has penetrated the anal lumen and stays in the anal canal during evacuation

the last degree of severity, of the phenomenon of invagination of the rectal wall [4]. In our opinion, different grades of severity can be distinguished. In the first grade, a fold can be seen in the rectal wall, deepening gradually during rectal evacuation to form an intussusception of the full thickness of the rectal wall protruding into the rectal lumen; this is called an *intrarectal intussusception* (Fig. 15.1). In the second grade, the apex of the rectal

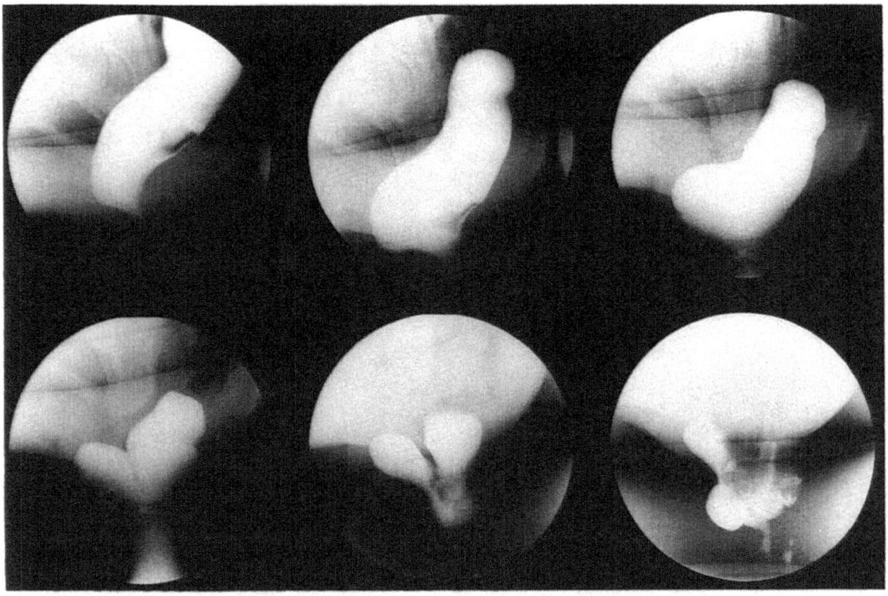

**Fig. 15.3.** Anterior wall infolding leading to the development of an intra-anal rectal intussusception

intussusception passes into the anal canal and remains in it during straining to form an *intra-anal rectal intussusception* (Figs. 15.2–15.4). In the third grade, the intussusception passes through the anal canal to form an *external rectal prolapse* (Fig. 15.5). In some patients, this process develops gradually and slowly (Fig. 15.5) so that it is easy to recognise. In other patients, the rectal wall prolapses suddenly, only at the end of rectal evacuation, so that it is essential to ask the patient to empty the rectum completely during examination [5]. The external rectal prolapse can be either spontaneously reducible when the patient ceases to strain or only manually reducible by digital manoeuvre.

Loss of the normal way in which the rectum fits into the sacral curve has been noted in complete rectal prolapse [6]. The rectum takes up a vertical course, displaced away from the sacral curve, which can be shown on the film taken when the patient is straining [7]. When there is an increased distance between the sacrum and the rectum, this indicates the presence of a mesorectum, which may facilitate full rectal wall intussusception [8].

In cases of intra-anal rectal intussusception, the intussusception occludes the anal canal, preventing further evacuation of rectal contents. Therefore, the most common symptom is terminal constipation, except if the anal sphincter has been forced, which leads paradoxically to a variable degree of incontinence. This latter condition is frequently associated with external rectal prolapse, especially when it has existed for a long time.

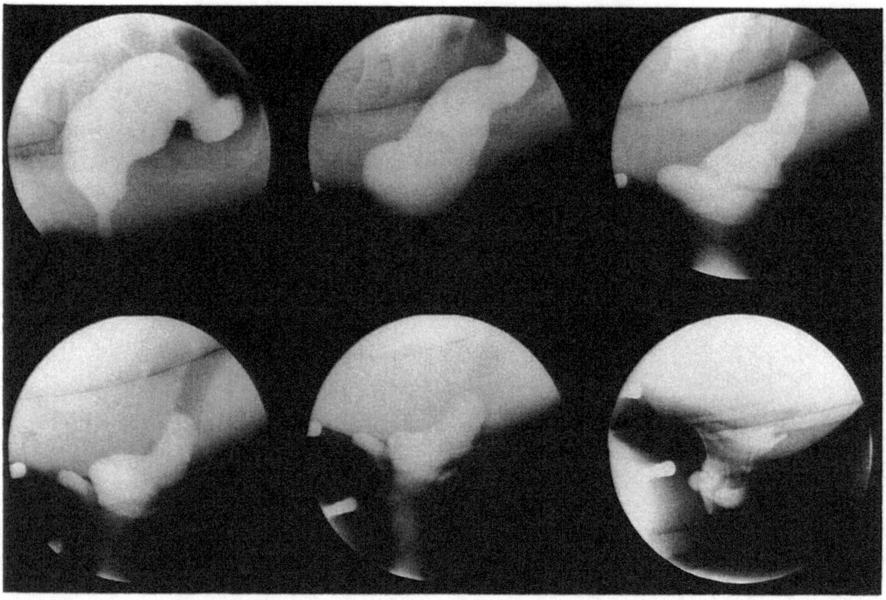

**Fig. 15.4.** Circumferential infolding leading to an intra-anal rectal intussusception at strain

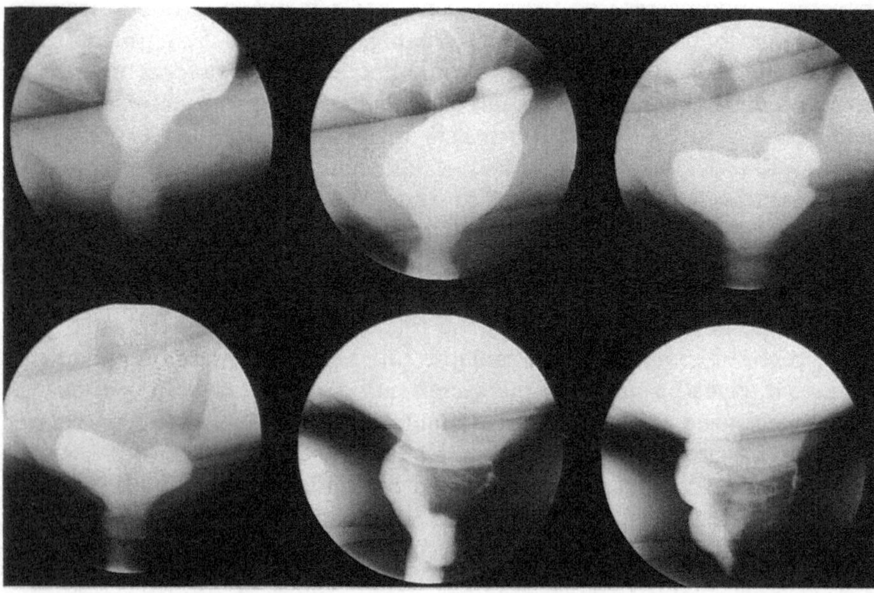

**Fig. 15.5.** Slow development of an external rectal prolapse during straining

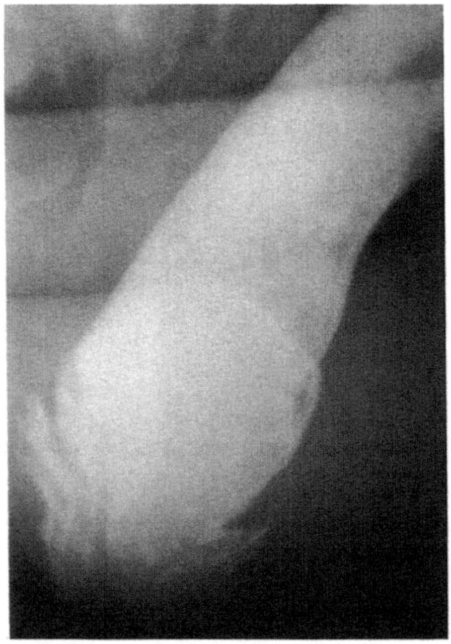

**Fig. 15.6.** Mucosal distal intrarectal intussusception. Only the mucosal part (<5 mm width) of the rectal wall is involved in the intussusception, which starts from the lower end of the rectum

There is usually no doubt regarding the clinical diagnosis of complete rectal prolapse. Lesser stages can, however, give rise to diagnostic difficulties. The physician or the patient and especially the young patient) may fail to realise that prolapse is occurring, or the patient may be too embarrassed to admit to his condition spontaneously. In our experience, of 32 patients presenting external rectal prolapse, only 14 had mentioned it in the anamnesis [9].

*Mucosal Intussusception.* In some cases, the intussusception starts as a mucosal folding which measures up to 5 mm in width and may stay like that (Fig. 15.6). When the fold increases in thickness, this implies a full-thickness rectal intussusception measuring more than 5 mm in width [10] (Fig. 15.1).

*Associated Enterocele.* When the patient presents a deep pouch of Douglas, which has been considered a predisposing factor to conditions such as long mesorectum and redundancy of the sigmoid colon, intestinal or sigmoid loops may be enclosed in the anterior wall of the rectal prolapse to form an enterocele. This condition can be suspected on radiographs when the anterior wall is abnormally thick, when it contains air bubbles or when there have been previously opacified intestinal loops.

*Level of Intussusception Formation.* In a series of 95 cases of intussusception, Mahieu et al. [9] observed that 60% originated from the anterior rectal wall (Fig. 15.3) and 32% from an annular segment of the rectal wall (Fig.

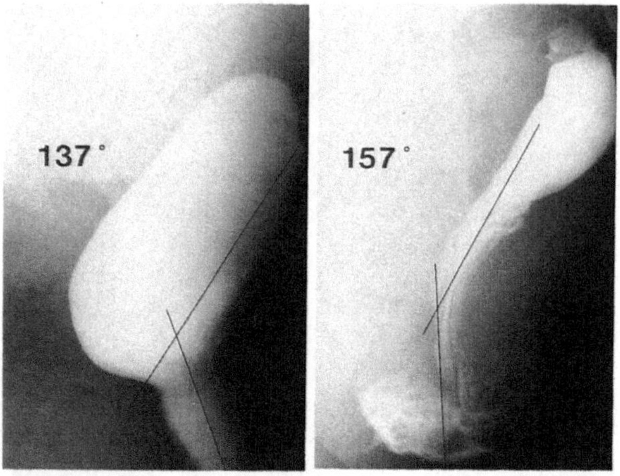


**Fig. 15.7.** Abnormal widening of the anorectal angle at strain in a patient presenting an external rectal prolapse (*right*) in comparison with a normal subject under the same conditions (*left*)

15.4). The posterior wall was very rarely the origin of intussusception. Intussusception most often develops at the level of a Houston valve, at 6–8 cm from the anal margin [11]: this is a proximal intussusception (Fig. 15.1). In three of the author's cases, prolapse originated from the rectal region located immediately above the anal canal, confirming observations made by others [3]: this is a distal intussusception (Fig. 15.6). Defaecography has demonstrated that the anorectal angle only becomes significantly higher when an intussusception passes the upper edge of the puborectalis, to lie intra- or extra-anally [5] (Fig. 15.7).

*Findings After Rectopexy*. In 20 patients who had undergone Orr-Loygue rectopexy (usually for external rectal prolapse), easy evacuation of the distal rectum was observed whereas a residue remained in the proximal part even after repeated straining efforts. Terminal constipation, a frequent complaint of these operated patients, is probably related to this observation.

### *15.1.2 Solitary Ulcer Syndrome of the Rectum*

#### *15.1.2.1 Introduction*

Solitary ulcer syndrome of the rectum (SUSR) is a chronic benign condition that mainly affects young adults and is characterised by the passage of blood and mucus per rectum, pain and persistent straining, often with a feeling of anal blockage. The condition was first described by Cruveilheir in 1870, and in 1969 Madigan and Morson first reviewed the condition extensively on the

**Table 15.1.** Presenting symptoms in 43 patients with SUSR

| | No. | % |
|---|---|---|
| Bleeding | 36 | 88 |
| Stool frequency and tenesmus | 37 | 86 |
| Mucous discharge | 34 | 79 |
| Lower abdominal or perineal pain | 26 | 60 |
| Straining at stool | 21 | 49 |
| Feeling of anal blockage | 14 | 33 |
| Self-digitation | 9 | 21 |
| Incontinence | 5 | 12 |

basis of 68 patients [12]. The term "solitary ulcer" is misleading because the ulcers can be solitary or multiple, or there can be no mucosal ulceration.
In 1975, Rutter and Riddel [13] reported that the majority of patients with SUSR strain at stool and established a clear connection between excessive straining and ulceration of the rectal mucosa. The diagnosis is usually based on clinical findings, sigmoidoscopy or barium enema (preferably double contrast) and on examination of rectal biopsy specimens. Defaecography is of special interest when this condition is suspected.

### *15.1.2.2 Clinical Findings*

In a series of 43 patients presenting SUSR [14] (Table 15.1), 27 were female and 16 male. Their ages ranged from 16 to 56 years, with a mean of 33. The most common symptoms were bleeding (88%), frequency of defaecation and tenesmus (86%) and mucous discharge (79%). Straining at stool was related by 49% of the patients. With regard to the latter finding, it has been reported that patients with SUSR spend a lot of time – average: 33 min – at stool each day [15].
A feeling of anal blockage was mentioned by a third of the patients and self-digitation by a fifth of them. Some patients feel that they are pushing a blockage out of the way to enable evacuation to progress normally, while others feel that they are digitally evacuating their bowels. In cases of intra-anal rectal intussusception, the proximal rectal wall intussuscepts into the lumen of the distal rectum, blocking the anal canal during straining and leading to a vicious cycle of incomplete evacuation and repeated straining [16].
The degree of bleeding is usually relatively minor, although some authors relate that major haemorrhage, requiring multiple blood transfusions, can occur [12, 17].
The duration of symptoms prior to the diagnosis of SUSR is usually long, an average 5–6 years [17].

### *15.1.2.3 Endoscopic and Histopathological Findings*

Typically, proctoscopy reveals a solitary, benign-appearing ulcer with discrete, slightly raised margins on the anterior or anterolateral wall of the rectum 7–10 cm from the anal verge [12, 13]. However, multiple ulcers are present in 25%–30% of cases [12], the location is occasionally the posterior or lateral wall of the rectum, and the distance from the anal verge may vary between 3 and 15 cm [12, 14]. Other patients may present localised proctitis with a nodular or erythematous mucosa, but no ulcers [12, 13].
As we have seen, SUSR is an uncommon condition with a variety of endoscopic findings. The diagnosis is therefore usually based on findings of rectal biopsy rather than on the gross appearance at proctoscopy. It should be recognised that a definitive diagnosis of SUSR can be made on histological criteria [12], regardless of the presence or absence of ulceration [17]. These histological criteria have been described by Madigan and Morson and are pathognomonic for the condition [12].

### *15.1.2.4 Radiographic Findings*

*Barium Enema.* One or more abnormality is usually found on double contrast enema (Table 15.2). The most common finding is thickening of the rectal folds (Figs. 15.8, 15.9). Rectal spasm is often present, being expressed by an immediate contraction of the rectal ampulla after air insufflation. The thickening of the folds can be diffuse (Fig. 15.9), nodular or pseudopolypoid (Fig. 15.10) and sometimes suggests a tumour (Fig. 15.11). Ulceration can be solitary or multiple, and located either on the anterior rectal wall or laterally. Granularity seems to be the expression of a non-ulcerative phase presenting intense fibrosis in the submucosa [9]. Rectal stricture is seldom. Radiologically, the rectal ampulla is never strictly normal in the author's experience, but this opinion is not shared by all authors [15, 18].
The differential diagnosis of SUSR includes granulomatous, ulcerative, traumatic, ischaemic, post-radiation or drug-induced proctitis, lymphogranuloma

**Fig. 15.8** (*upper left*). Solitary ulcer syndrome of the rectum. Barium enema showed thickening of the rectal folds and distal valve of Houston. Defaecography revealed intra-anal rectal intussusception ▶

**Fig. 15.9** (*upper right*). Solitary ulcer syndrome of the rectum. Defaecography showed external rectal prolapse

**Fig. 15.10** (*lower left*). Solitary ulcer syndrome of the rectum. Pseudopolypoid changes in the rectal mucosa. Defaecography showed external rectal prolapse

**Fig. 15.11** (*lower right*). Solitary ulcer syndrome of the rectum. Mucosal ulcerations and fold thickening may simulate a tumour. Defaecography showed external rectal prolapse

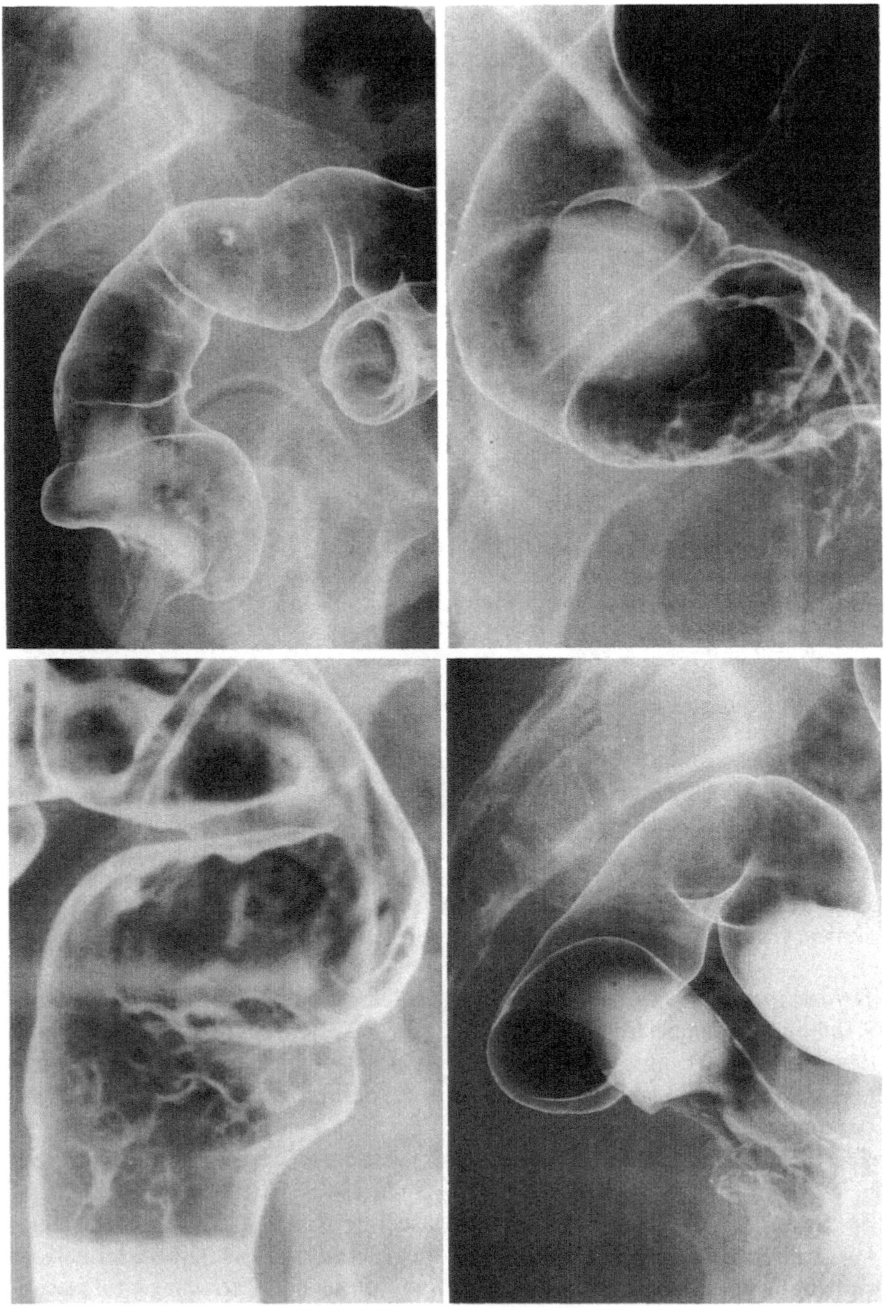

**Table 15.2.** Radiological findings on double contrast enema in 33 patients with SUSR

| | No. | % |
|---|---|---|
| Thickening of rectal folds | 26 | 79 |
| Rectal spasm | 24 | 73 |
| Ulceration | 16 | 48 |
| Nodular, pseudopolypoid or pseudotumoral mucosal folds | 9 | 27 |
| Granularity | 2 | 6 |
| Rectal stricture | 2 | 6 |
| Normal | 0 | 0 |

**Table 15.3.** Findings at defaecography ($n$ = 80) in SUSR

| Findings | No. | % |
|---|---|---|
| 1. Intussusception and prolapse | 66 | 83 |
| a) External rectal prolapse | 27 | 34 |
| b) Intra-anal | 19 | 24 |
| c) Intrarectal | 20 | 25 |
| 2. Pelvic floor descent at rest | 22 | 27.5 |
| 3. Pelvic floor descent at strain | 17 | 21 |
| 4. Wide opening of the anal canal | 12 | 15 |
| 5. Rectocele | 4 | 5 |
| 6. Dyskinaesia of the puborectalis | 4 | 5 |
| 7. Mucosal prolapse | 3 | 4 |
| 8. Normal | 1 | 1 |

venereum, amoebic proctocolitis, and benign or malignant tumour. The clinical history is often helpful in differentiating these conditions.

*Defaecography*. Detection of radiological abnormalities on barium enema is helpful in suggesting the diagnosis. In addition, it justifies performing defaecography to investigate the underlying mechanism causing the mucosal lesion. Table 15.3 reports the findings at defaecography in a series of 80 patients.

The most frequent abnormality was the presence of an intussusception, seen in 83% of the 80 patients. Of these, 27 (34%) had an external rectal prolapse, 19 (24%) an intra-anal intussusception and 20 (25%) an intrarectal intussusception. Intussusceptions of the rectum are usually described as starting in the midrectal region; thus they are usually proximal intussusceptions. However, we have seen cases in which intussusception commenced just above the anorectal junction (distal intussusceptions) [9].

Constant or transient dyskinetic contraction of the puborectalis and the pelvic floor (Fig. 15.12) was recognised in only four cases (5%). Excessive

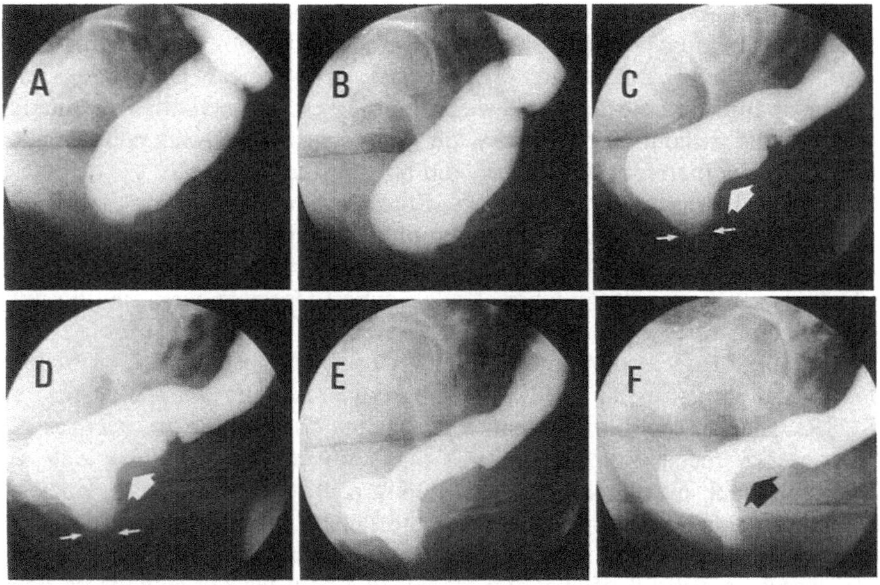


**Fig. 15.12A-F.** Dyskinaesia of the puborectalis (*arrows*); the muscle is contracted during rectal evacuation instead of being relaxed, resulting in incomplete emptying of the rectal contents

pelvic floor descent was noted in 22 patients (27%) at rest and in 17 (21%) at strain. Rectocele was recognised in four patients (5%), while three (4%) had prolapse of the rectal wall mucosa.

Caution must be exercised in interpreting defaecograms as a study on 47 healthy young volunteers showed that a degree of perineal descent, rectocele and even intussusception can occur in asymptomatic subjects [2] (see also Chap. 6). It is therefore not to be forgotten that while defaecography can show abnormalities, reliance should not be placed on these results alone, and confirmation should be sought by other techniques, as well as by correlation with clinical findings.

### *15.1.2.5 Aetiopathological Hypothesis Related to the Results of Defaecography*

The pathogenesis of SUSR is uncertain and several theories have been proposed to account for the clinical and histological changes seen in this syndrome. From electromyographic studies it has been suggested that there is a functional disorder, a dyscoordination of the pelvic floor muscles, in particular hypertonia of the puborectalis during defaecation, leading to difficulty in rectal evacuation [13]. This can be easily observed on defaecography

as an increase in the imprint of the puborectalis on the posterior wall of the anorectal junction [9]. In our series only a few patients showed this feature; thus many patients with SUSR have no dyskinetic puborectalis on defaecography and, furthermore, we have observed patients with a dyskinetic puborectalis without SUSR. From the radiological standpoint puborectalis dyskinaesia is therefore uncommon and not specific for SUSR.
Trauma to the rectal wall or the apex of the rectal intussusception, occurring spontaneously [19] or due to self-digitation or instrumentation [20], has been suggested as a cause of SUSR. However, many patients without solitary ulcer who perform self-digitation, for example those with rectocele, do not cause trauma to the rectum.
The results of defaecography indicate a close relationship between SUSR and rectal intussusception (the latter being present in 79% of cases of SUSR). Intussusception may lead to ischaemia due to pressure necrosis of the anterior rectal wall caused by it being forced into the upper end of the anal canal and pinched by an actively contracting external sphincter. Fibrosis and muscular hypertrophy in the lamina propria, obliterating the mucosal capillaries, and stretching and rupture of submucosal vessels might also occur as a result of shearing movements between the submucosa and mucosa. Rutter [21] has discussed the possibility that mucosal prolapse starting as a proximal or a distal intussusception may be the first step in the development of SUSR. It has been postulated that repeated straining causes occult prolapse of the anterior wall of the rectum with ulceration of the prolapsed mucosa due to mechanical trauma and/or ischaemia. This theory would explain why ulceration is typically found on the anterior rectal wall. The causative role of rectal intussusception or prolapse is supported by the healing of the rectal lesions observed after rectopexy.

#### *15.1.2.6 Treatment*

For the patients without prolapse or intussusception, and perhaps even for the others, education about bowel habits, with avoidance of straining at stool and the institution of a high fibre diet, should be the main line of approach. SUSR invariably seems difficult to treat, even if rectopexy relieves many of the symptoms related to the occult or overt prolapse.

#### *15.1.2.7 Conclusion*

Clinical history, endoscopy and barium enema can help in suggesting the diagnosis of SUSR. Histopathology is usually characteristic and rectal biopsy is essential to establish firmly the existence of the condition. Defaecography is the investigation of choice in that it shows the underlying functional disorder and can help in selecting patients for surgery.

## 15.2 Prolapse and Enterocele: The Surgeon's View

J.H.C. Kuijpers

The pelvic floor muscle forms the bottom of the abdominal cavity. It contains the sphincters of the bladder and colon and supports the abdominal organs. Functionally the muscle can be subdivided into the external anal sphincter, the puborectalis sling and the levator ani muscle. It has a funnel-like configuration. The levator ani muscle forms the upper, broader part of the funnel, and the external anal sphincter, the lower, smaller part. The angle that creates the shape of the funnel is caused by the puborectalis sling [22, 23]. This angle can be measured by calculating the angle between the axis of the rectum and anal canal, the anorectal angle [22].

The muscle is always in a state of slight contraction, even at rest or during sleep, which is in contrast with most other striated muscles. It therefore can immediately and reflexively react to increases in intra-abdominal pressure by further contraction and thus maintain faecal continence. The radiological manifestation of this slight contraction at rest is an anorectal angle of about 90° due to the horizontal course of the rectal axis.

Denervation of the pelvic floor muscle leads to impaired function. Sphincter contraction is reduced, which will lead to urinary or faecal incontinence, or both. Moreover, as a result of impaired puborectalis contraction the anorectal angle increases to about 135° due to the more vertical course of the rectal axis [23, 24]. This gives less support to the bladder and rectum, which, instead of leaning *on* the pelvic floor, will start to slide down *from* it, bulge outwards and prolapse. The centre of the pelvic floor descends in relation to the bony pelvic structures; ligaments elongate, structures widen, and septa get thinner. The pouch of Douglas is deepened; it splits the rectovaginal septum proximally and exposes the anterior rectal and posterior vaginal wall to the abdominal pressure. If time permits, prolapse of both walls is a logical consequence, resulting in an enterocele (Fig. 15.13) and anterior rectal wall prolapse (Fig. 15.14), or even complete rectal prolapse. The faecal stream is not stopped by the pelvic floor muscle but only diverted and subsequently directed anteriorly at the distal rectovaginal septum, which will give way and bulge outwards, creating a rectocele (Fig. 15.15).

Small cystoceles, enteroceles and rectoceles are common findings in older females and only need treatment when they become symptomatic. Complete rectal prolapse needs treatment because the prolapse is inconvenient, embarrassing and painful, and causes continence disorders. More than 200 different operative procedures to treat complete rectal prolapse have been reported in the surgical literature, which makes selection of the best procedure difficult [25, 26]. The treatment concepts are usually based on abnormalities of local anatomy that are commonly found in patients with complete rectal prolapse, such as a deep cul-de-sac of Douglas, a patulous and lax anal sphincter, a redundant rectosigmoid, insufficient pelvic floor

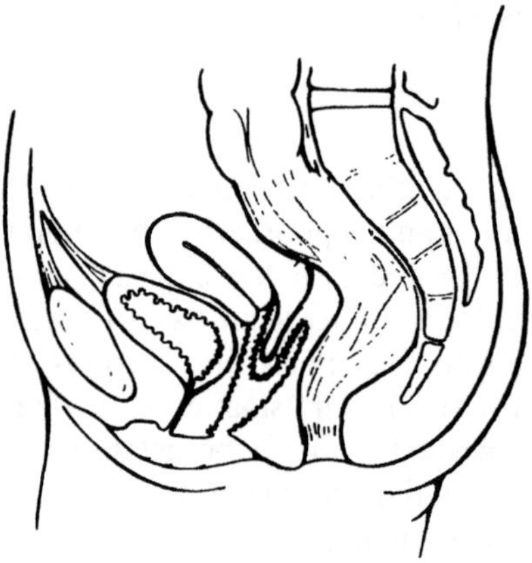

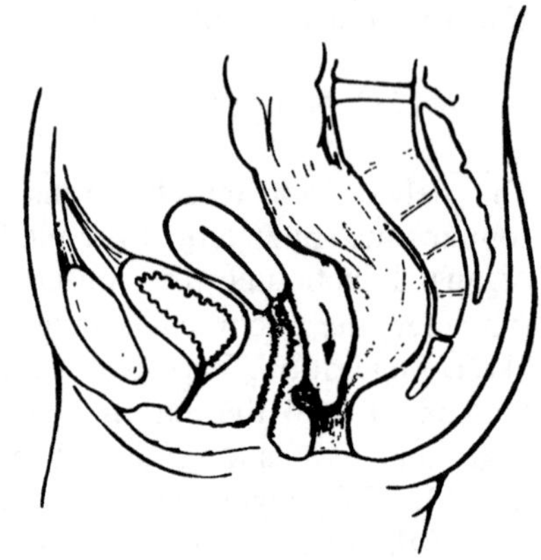

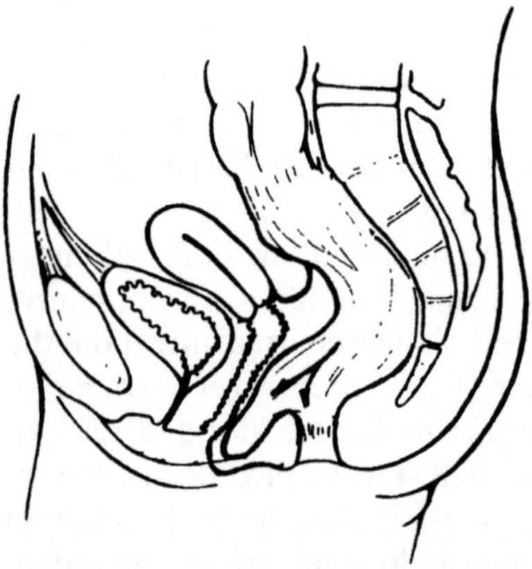

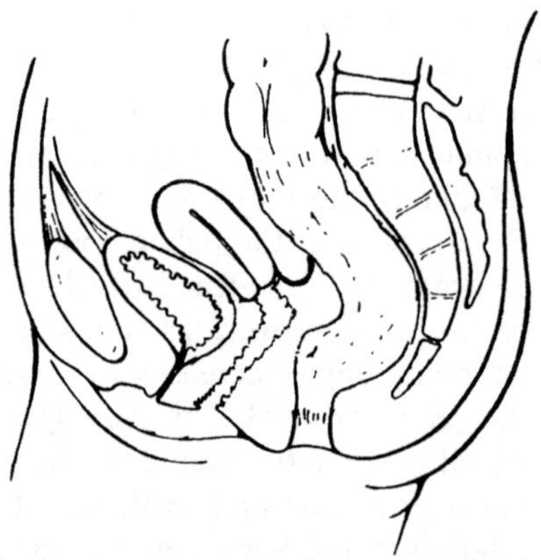

**Fig. 15.13** (*upper left*). Development of an enterocele due to exposure of the posterior vaginal wall to the abdominal pressure following proximal splitting of the rectovaginal septum by the pouch of Douglas

**Fig. 15.14** (*upper right*). Development of anterior rectal wall prolapse due to exposure of the wall to the abdominal pressure following proximal splitting of the rectovaginal septum by the pouch of Douglas

**Fig. 15.15** (*lower left*). Redirection of the faecal stream towards the distal rectovaginal septum. A rectocele is created when the septum gives way and bulges outwards

**Fig. 15.16** (*lower right*). The Douglas pouch after rectopexy

function, rectal intussusception or lack of fascial support of the rectum against the sacrum. All concepts of a etiology have been based on these observations, and the main argument has been about which of the abnormalities is cause and which effect. The options for therapy included obliteration of the peritoneal pouch of Douglas, narrowing of the anal canal, restoration of the pelvic floor, resection of the abundant bowel by either an abdominal or a perineal approach, and suspension or fixation of the rectum to the sacrum or other structures by the abdominal, perineal or transsacral route [25, 26]. Good results have been reported from newly introduced procedures, but most of these operations have not given good lasting results in the hands of other surgeons.

Critical study and comparison of the different surgical techniques shows that the best results are obtained by procedures that, whether or not they are combined with some other procedure, fixate the rectum to the sacrum. It is therefore now commonly accepted that complete rectal prolapse is an intussusception of the rectum which is caused by inadequate or loose sacral fixation.

Another, more sophisticated way of deciding which procedure to employ is based on the application of the colorectal laboratory, a collection of colorectal and anorectal functional tests that have been developed to study the function of the different parts of the mechanism of continence [27, 28].

Defaecography, the technique for the radiological visualisation of defaecation, is the preferred means of studying rectal and pelvic floor function [24, 28–32]. It enables us to determine whether the presumed causative dysfunction on which the operative procedure is based indeed exists. Furthermore, it establishes whether the surgical procedure performed has completely corrected the dysfunction and eliminated the mechanism of prolapse, and whether any new functional or anatomical disorders have been created by the procedure [32]. It should be pointed out that in the past little or no attention has been paid to whether all the rectal narrowing, wrapping, suspending, fixing, encircling, plicating and even resecting involved in the various procedures can be performed without affecting rectal function, or rather faecal continence, which is already severely impaired in most patients. Addition of a small bowel barium study will reveal the presence of an enterocele.

Defaecographic studies have confirmed that complete rectal prolapse is an intussusception of the rectum [28–32]. They have demonstrated tht it starts as a prolapse of the anterior rectal wall a few centimetres from the anal canal, followed by a posterior rectal wall prolapse creating an intussusception into the lower rectum and subsequently into the anal canal. Marked inferior and anterior descent of the rectum from the sacral concavity occurs, and finally, the intussusception protrudes through the anal canal, forming a complete rectal prolapse.

It has also been demonstrated in a study comparing the results of defaecography performed before and after posterior rectopexy, that the procedure adequately corrected the radiological abnormalities without creating new ones. Rectal fixation was excellent and the configuration of the anterior and posterior rectal wall remained straight during straining. Posterior rectopexy is therefore a suitable procedure for the treatment of rectal prolapse [32, 33].

It may be concluded that an advocation of new surgical techniques for the treatment of complete rectal prolapse should be based not only on a low recurrence and complication rate, but also on results of tests that evaluate the effect of the procedure on faecal continence.

Posterior rectopexy is the simplest abdominal approach to the treatment of rectal prolapse. It involves thorough mobilisation and upward fixation of the rectum. The goal of rectal fixation is to keep the rectum attached in the desired "pulled-up" position until adequate fixation by scar tissue is achieved. This scar tissue is the explanation for its high success rate. Discussion nowadays focuses on how far the rectum should be mobilised, which, if any, foreign material should be used for rectal fixation, how it should be placed and whether colonic resection should be added.

The pouch of Douglas plays a crucial role in rectal prolapse (Fig. 15.16). As mentioned above, rectal prolapse starts as a prolapse of the anterior rectal wall, the peritoneal side of which is called the pouch of Douglas. When the anterior rectal wall protrudes outside the anal canal, it means that the pouch of Douglas, too, is below the perineal level. It is therefore essential to bring the pouch of Douglas up as high as possible, preferably to the level of the cervix so that the split septum is restored, and to fixate the pulled-up rectum at the corresponding level. In so doing, the distance between the pouch of Douglas and the perineum is maximised, which is the best way to prevent a recurrence. When the rectum is pulled up tightly, stretching the lateral ligaments, and the pouch of Douglas is still situated below the level of the cervix, thus exposing the posterior vaginal wall to the abdominal pressure, division of the lateral ligaments will bring the pouch of Douglas up further. If a deep pouch of Douglas persists despite adequate posterior and lateral mobilisation, the peritoneum covering it should be removed, in so doing fixing the anterior rectal wall to the posterior vaginal wall by scar tissue and reconstructing the split rectovaginal septum. It is obvious that preoperative investigation for the presence of an enterocele is not indicated since a coexistent enterocele will in any case be cured by this procedure. The level of the pouch of Douglas thus plays a critical role in the adequacy of rectal mobilisation and the efficacy of the procedure.

In the research laboratory, defaecography has proven to be a suitable and valuable test in studying the mechanism of complete rectal prolapse. As already mentioned, it has demonstrated that complete rectal prolapse is a rectal intussusception and that posterior rectopexy adequately corrects the intussusception and cures the prolapse without creating new anatomical or functional disorders, which makes it the procedure of choice for this condition. The diagnostic value of defaecography, however, is limited. Surgery is always indicated when a complete rectal prolapse is diagnosed, and selection of the surgical technique to be performed is still based on personal experience and preference and not on defaecographic data. Moreover, the coexistence of an enterocele does not influence the selection of a procedure since it will be cured anyway. Defaecography is therefore indicated only to evaluate a prolapse of unknown origin.

## References


1. Ekberg O, Mahieu PHG, Bartram C, Piloni V (1990) Defaecography: dynamic radiological imaging in proctology. Gastroenterol Int 3:53–69
2. Shorvon PJ, McHugh S, Diamant NE, Somers S, Stevenson GW (1989) Defecography in normal volunteers: results and implications. Gut 30:1737–1749
3. Broden B, Snellman B (1968) Procidentia of the rectum studied with cineradiography: a contribution to the discussion of causative mechanism. Dis Colon Rectum 11:330–347
4. Mahieu PHG, Pringot J, Vanheuverzwyn R, Goncette L (1981) Les prolapsus du rectum: apport du lavement et de la défécographie. Acta Gastroenterol Belg 44:502–512
5. Mahieu PHG, Pringot J and Bodart P (1984) Defecography: I. Description of a new procedure and results in normal patients. Gastrointest Radiol 9:247–251
6. Ripstein CB and Lanter B (1963) Etiology and surgical therapy of massive prolapse of the rectum. Ann Surg 157:259–264
7. Ripstein CB (1965) Surgical care of massive rectal prolapse. Dis Colon Rectum 8:34–38
8. Ripstein CB (1952) Treatment of massive rectal prolapse. Am J Surg 83:68–71
9. Mahieu PHG, Pringot J and Bodart P (1984) Defecography: II. Contribution to the diagnosis of defecation disorders. Gastrointest Radiol 9:253–261
10. Mahieu PHG (1988) Defecography: a radiological method for evaluation of anorectal disorders. In Margulis AR, Burhenne HJ (eds) Alimentary tract roentgenology (2 vols). Mosby, St Louis, pp 933–941
11. Bartram Cl, Mahieu PHG (1985) Radiology of the pelvic floor. In: Henry M, Swash M (eds) Coloproctology and the pelvic floor. Butterworths, London, pp 151–186
12. Madigan MR, Morson BC (1969) Solitary ulcer of the rectum. Gut 10:871–881
13. Rutter KRP, Riddell RH (1975) Solitary ulcer syndrome of the rectum. Clin Gastroenterol 4:505–530
14. Mahieu PHG (1986) Barium enema and defaecography in the diagnosis and evaluation of the solitary rectal ulcer syndrome. Int J Colorect Dis 1:85–90
15. Mackle EJ, Manton Mills JO and Parks TG (1990) The investigation of anorectal dysfunction in the solitary rectal ulcer syndrome. Int J Colorect Dis 5:21–24
16. Goei R, Baeten C, Arends J (1988) Solitary rectal ulcer syndrome: findings at barium enema study and defecography. Radiology 168:303–306
17. Levine MS, Piccolello ML, Sollenberger LC, Laufer I, Saul SH (1986) Solitary rectal ulcer syndrome: a radiological diagnosis? Gastrointest Radiol 11:187–193
18. Feczko PJ, O'Connell DJ, Riddell RH, Frank PH (1980) Solitary rectal ulcer syndrome: radiologic manifestations. AJR 135:499-506
19. Schweiger M, Alexander-Williams J (1977) Solitary ulcer syndrome of the rectum. Its association with occult rectal prolapse. Lancet 1:170–171
20. Thomson H and Hill D (1980) Solitary rectal ulcer: always a self-induced condition? Br J Surg 67:784–785
21. Rutter KRP (1985) Solitary ulcer syndrome of the rectum: its relation to mucosal prolapse. In: Henry M, Swash M (eds) Coloproctology and the pelvic floor. Butterworths, London, pp 282–298
22. Kuijpers JHC (1990) Anatomy and physiology of the rectum. Neth J Med 37:S2–S5
23. Kuijpers JHC, Scheuer M (1990) Disorders of impaired faecal control: a clinical and manometric study. Dis Colon Rectum 33:207–211
24. Mahieu P, Pringot J, Bodart P (1984) Defecography I. Description of a new procedure and results in normal patients. Gastrointest Radiol 9:247–251

25. Kuijpers JHC (1992) Surgery on rectal prolapse. In: Progress in pelvic surgery. World J Surg (to be published)
26. Wassef R, Rothenberger D, Goldberg S (1986) Rectal prolapse. Curr Probl Surg XXIII
27. Kuijpers JHC (1988) Diagnosis and treatment of defecation disorders. Scand J Gastroenterol 23 [Suppl 154]:72–76
28. Smith LE: Practical guide to anorectal testing 1st edn. Ikagu-Shon, New York
29. Kuijpers JHC, Strijk S (1984) Diagnosis of disturbances of continence and defaecation. Dis Colon Rectum 27:658–662
30. Broden B, Snellman B (1968) Procidentia of the rectum studied with cineradiography: a contribution to the discussion of causative mechanism. Dis Colon Rectum 11:330–347
31. Bartolo DCC, Bartram C, Kuijpers JHC, Mahieu PHG, Stevenson G, Fork FT, Womack N, Kodner I (1988) Symposium on proctography. Int J Colorectal Dis 3:67–83
32. Kuijpers JHC, DeMorre H (1988) Towards a selection of the most appropriate procedure in the treatment of complete rectal prolapse. Dis Colon Rectum 31:355–357
33. Kuijpers JHC (1991) Cineproctography. Semin Colorectal Surg 3(2)

# 16 Rectal Outpocketing

R. Hauck

## 16.1 Introduction

The rectum, is easily accessible for digital examination, rectoscopy and endoscopy. Many of the outpocketings of the rectal wall are palpable at rest in the lithotomy position. What additional information of the position and shape of rectal outpocketings and their relationship to adjoining structures can be gained, then, by defaecography? Which examination technique is the most suitable?

### *16.1.1 Examination Technique*

We employ the examination technique described in Chap. 5. In our experience four steps are particularly important for the diagnosis of rectal outpocketings at rest and during defaecation:

1. Rotating fluoroscopy of the contrast medium-filled rectum in the standing position to detect lateral outpocketings. If the patient is examined only in the lateral projection, such outpocketings can be obscured by other structures in the same plane.
2. Observation of the evacuation capability of each consecutive segment of the rectum in order not to miss transient bends or folds.
3. Documentation of the evacuated rectum in the anterioposterior projection while the patient is straining.
4. Contrast of the anal cleft and the vagina using contrast medium paste and a contrast medium-soaked vaginal tampon.

### *16.1.2 Classification of Rectal Outpocketings*

We propose a classification of five types of rectal outpocketings according to location and relation to adjoining structures:

1. Rectocele as ventral outpocketing of the rectum with radiological differentiation of subtypes and combination with other alterations
2. Hernia-like outpocketings of the pelvic floor

3. Outpocketings with three-dimensional displacement of the rectum, including "intussusceptions"
4. Atypical dorsal outpocketings
5. Other rare variations

This classification excludes anal and rectovaginal fistulae, cicatrices, ulcers, tumour craters and displacements and transformations of the rectum by surgery.
Recent reports concern the frequency of alterations of the rectal wall [4, 14, 17]. The wide discrepancy in the data on, for example, the ordinary rectocele arises from differences in examination technique (digital, instrumental, x-ray or combined) and in criteria (outpocketings of more or less than 2 cm, complete/incomplete evacuation).

## 16.2 The Rectocele

A rectocele is defined as a "ventral outpocketing of the rectum wall with incomplete evacuation" [17]. Because of the high prevalence of rectoceles some authors consider them a "normal appearance" [17]. We found rectal outpocketings in 338 of 507 consecutive defaecographies, a frequency of 66.7%. Of these, 302 (89%) were ventral, 27 (8%) were lateral and ventral, and 10 (3%) were dorsal.

### *16.2.1 Radiological Differentiation of Subtypes*

#### *16.2.1.1 Rectoceles Associated with a Symmetrically Shortened Anal Canal*

The subtype of ordinary rectocele with a functioning pelvic floor and an only symmetrically shortened anal canal (Fig. 16.1) is fairly rare.

#### *16.2.1.2 Rectoceles Associated with Weakness of the Pelvic Floor*

More often, patients with rectoceles exhibit a difference of the height of the muscular pelvic floor, with the ventral portion significantly lower than the dorsal portion. In females the muscular pelvic floor is relatively weak ventral to the anal canal, so effective muscular resistance against evacuation pressure ventral to the anal canal is absent in many cases (Fig. 16.2).
In some cases an increase of traction of the puborectalis muscle with consequent impression of the rectum can be observed. Probably there is an increase of muscular resistance against intra-abdominal pressure. Complete rectal evacuation is not observed in this situation (Fig. 16.3). Mahieu supposes the presence of a muscular spasm [15]. An illustration is given by Bartram et al. [2].

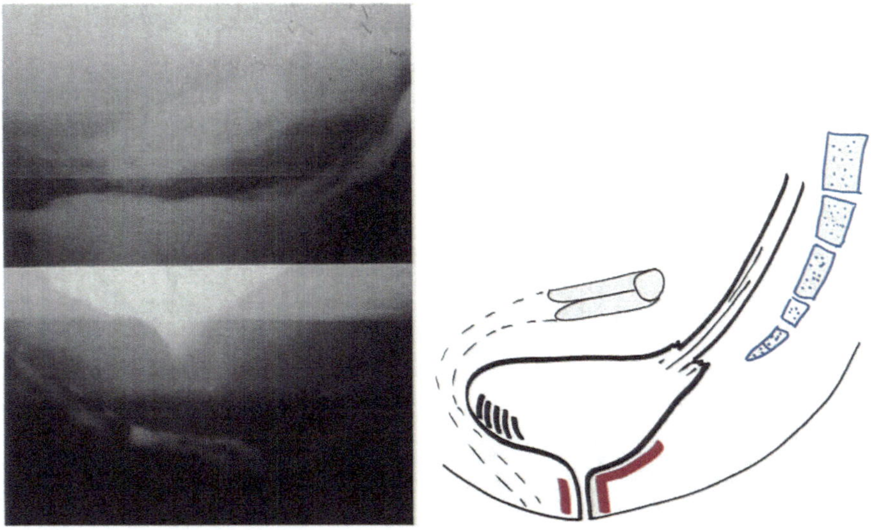

Fig. 16.1. Rectocele according to the common definition: weakening of rectovesical ligament, ventral outpocketing of rectum and shortening of anal canal in a 27-year-old woman. For key to colours, see p. 26

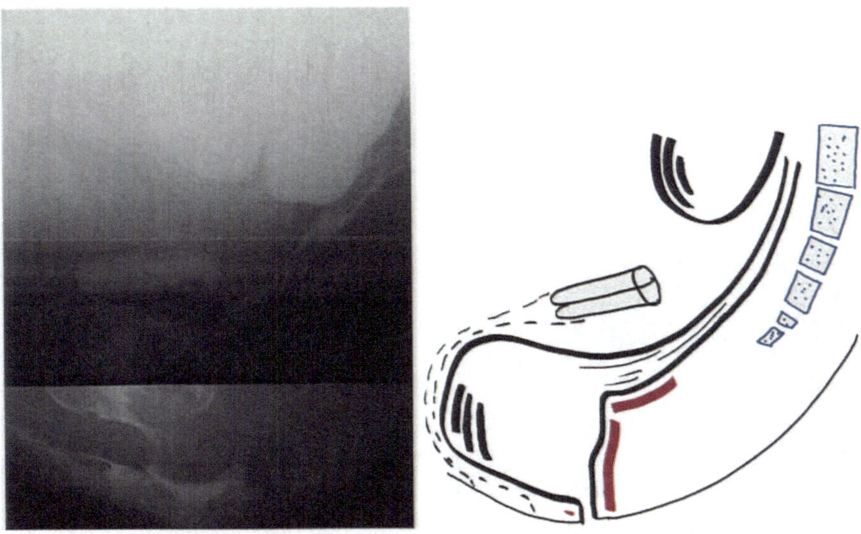

Fig. 16.2. Very frequent form of rectocele, characterized by different heights of anterior and posterior wall of anal canal. Remarkable involvement of vagina in a 24-year-old woman. About 82% of all rectoceles are of this type

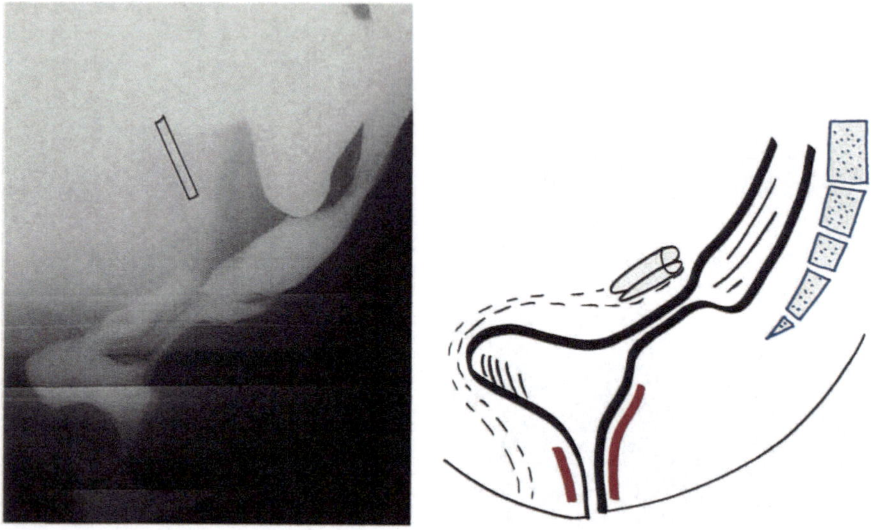

**Fig. 16.3.** Apparently spastic reaction of rectum together with rectocele in a 40-year-old woman. The frequency of this type is about 4%

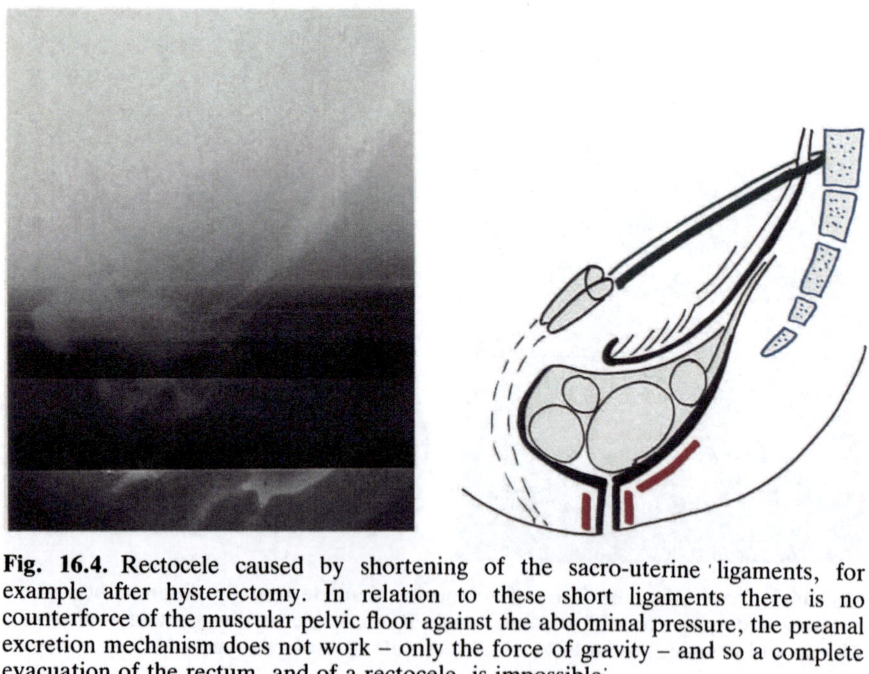

**Fig. 16.4.** Rectocele caused by shortening of the sacro-uterine ligaments, for example after hysterectomy. In relation to these short ligaments there is no counterforce of the muscular pelvic floor against the abdominal pressure, the preanal excretion mechanism does not work – only the force of gravity – and so a complete evacuation of the rectum, and of a rectocele, is impossible

Often a rectocele or inability to evacuate the rectum completely is accompanied by an obviously concentric decrease of the height of the pelvic floor (Fig. 16.4). Even though this kind of evacuation disorder is a rectocele according to the standard definition, it has a completely different cause. One reason for its development could be the weakness of the muscular pelvic floor – diagnosed digitally or by manometry – which cannot resist increasing intestinal pressure. Not infrequently, however, this kind of evacuation disorder can be observed after hysterectomy if the sacro-uterine ligaments had to be shortened and the fascia pelvis superior (see also Chap. 3) consequently allows only little excursion when intra-abdominal pressure increases. Pressure cannot be transmitted to the pelvic floor, and rectoceles bulge out between the pelvic floor and the fascia pelvis superior. Complete evacuation of the rectum is only possible with manual assistance.

#### *16.2.1.3 Rectoceles Combined with Enteroceles of Small Intestine or Colon*

Another subtype of rectocele does not occupy the outpocketing of the rectovaginal septum completely but becomes pushed into the excavation by an enterocele of the small or large intestine (Fig. 16.5). Partial evacuation is the result. In the lateral projection the squeezed rectocele is shaped like a tongue.

### *16.2.2 Excentric and Lateral Rectoceles*

Outpocketings of the rectum in excentric and lateral positions are also classified as rectoceles.
Regarding their pathological significance and their therapy, if any is necessary, they cannot be distinguished from the subtypes of rectocele described above. In the lateral projection a semitransparency of contrast medium retention is pathognomonic, as is overlapping of vaginal tampon and rectum contrast. (Fig. 16.6). Assessment of this phenomenon is possible only in the anterioposterior (a.p.) projection.

## 16.3 Hernias into the Gap of the Levator Ani Muscle

The levator ani muscle is aligned from the pelvic bone circumference in a funnel-like shape down towards the anal canal fixation. The muscle consists of several portions: Waldeyer [18] distinguished the pars anterior and the pars lateralis (Fig. 16.7). Between these parts of the muscle there is a region of decreased muscle diameter or even a fibrotic slot, the levator ani gap. Not infrequent are rectal outpocketings with herniation into this gap. Corresponding to the anterolateral alignment of the gap the outpocketings

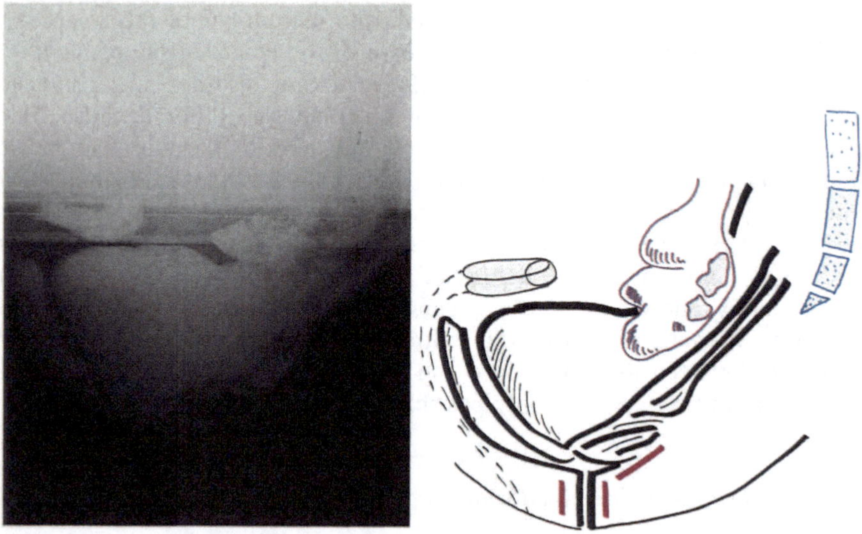

**Fig. 16.5.** Enormous enterocele containing small and large bowel in a 61-year-old woman 16 years after hysterectomy. Intestinal pressure acts via enterocele on a large rectocele squeezing out its contents. Routine digital examination can give the impression of a large rectocele apparently evacuated

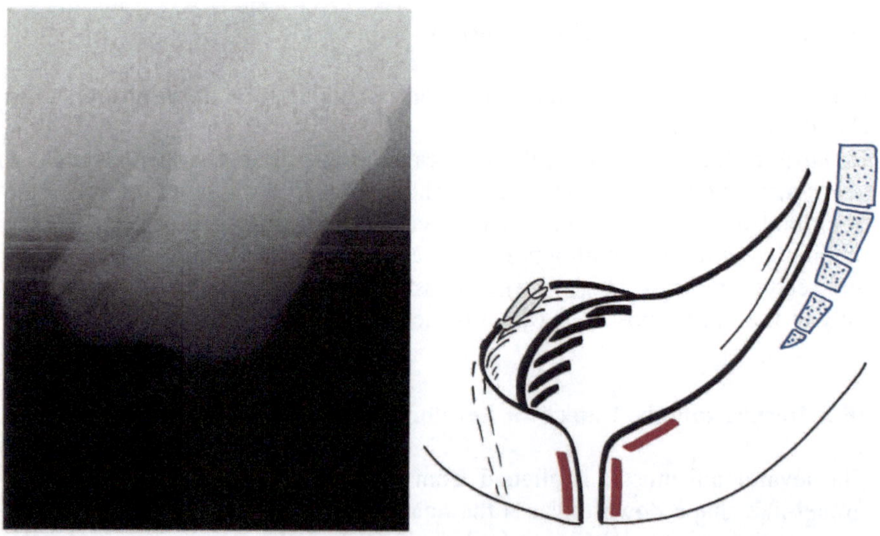

**Fig. 16.6.** Semilateral rectocele recognizable by half-shadowed aspect of distended rectum in a 67-year-old woman. **Fig. 16.6** continues on p. 151

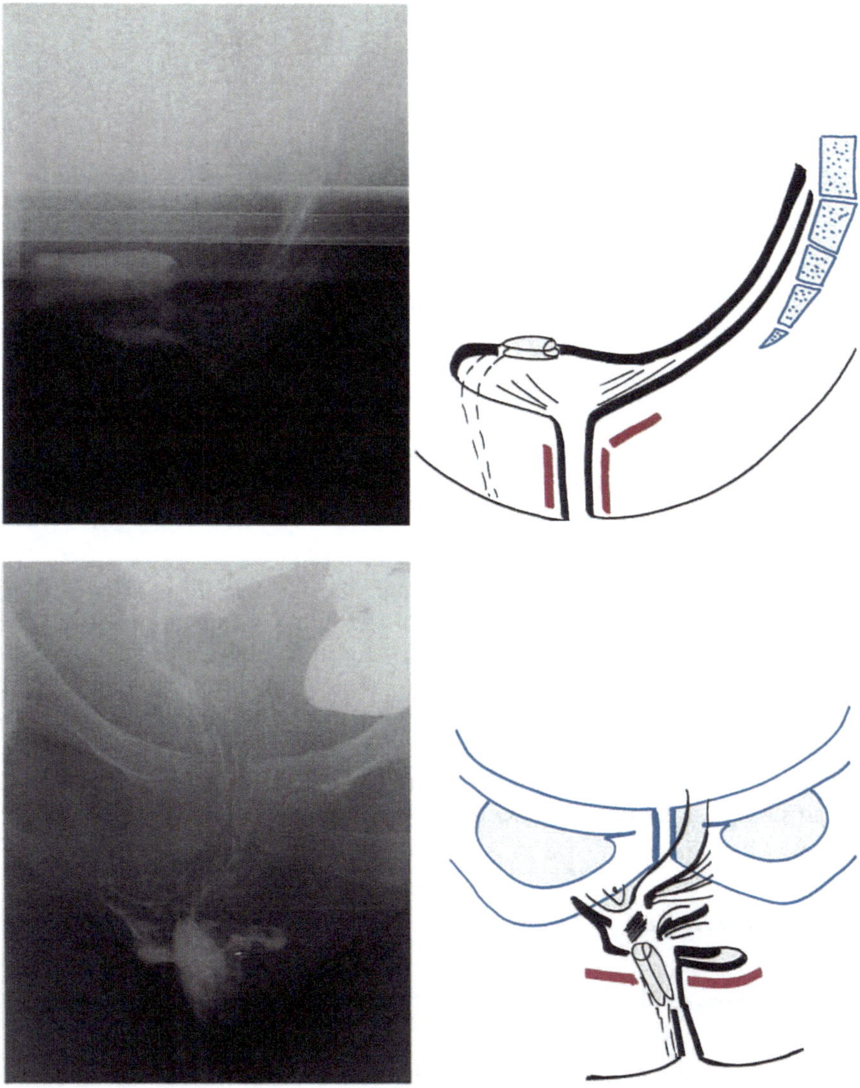

**Fig. 16.6.** *Above*: Evacuated bowel partly overshadows vaginal tampon. *Below*: The a.p. view clearly shows right lateral deviation of vagina which is more pronounced when rectum is full. The frequency of this finding is under 1% of all examinations

can be directed to the right or to the left side. This group of rectal disorder was found in 6% of all patients we examined. The hernia is mostly palpable in the sitting patient on defaecation. If a.p. screening and rotating fluoroscopy are carried out regularly, levator gap hernias can be identified easily. In the recent literature on defaecography there is no mention of this type of outpocketing.

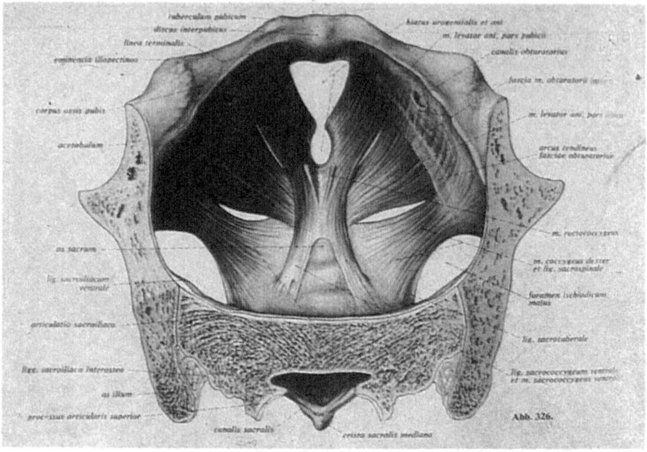


**Fig. 16.7.** The levator ani muscle [18]

In the case of hernia penetration through the levator ani gap the rectum contrast is behind the hernia contour in the lateral projection, so that the hernia contour is obscured. Compulsory for radiological diagnosis is a.p. fluoroscopy before or after evacuation. This kind of herniation can be overlooked easily when an a.p. view is not part of the standard examination programme.

In our experience 85% of herniations are to the left. No evident explanation for this bias can be derived from radiological findings.

### *16.3.1 Small Hernias*

#### *16.3.1.1 Hernias That Disappear on Evacuation*

Small hernias can normally be emptied on evacuation and are then no longer visible (Fig. 16.8).

#### *16.3.1.2 Hernias Unaltered by Evacuation*

Hernias with a diameter of approximately 2–3 cm may remain consistent in shape, position and size during evacuation (Fig. 16.9). In most cases they are of no clinical relevance.

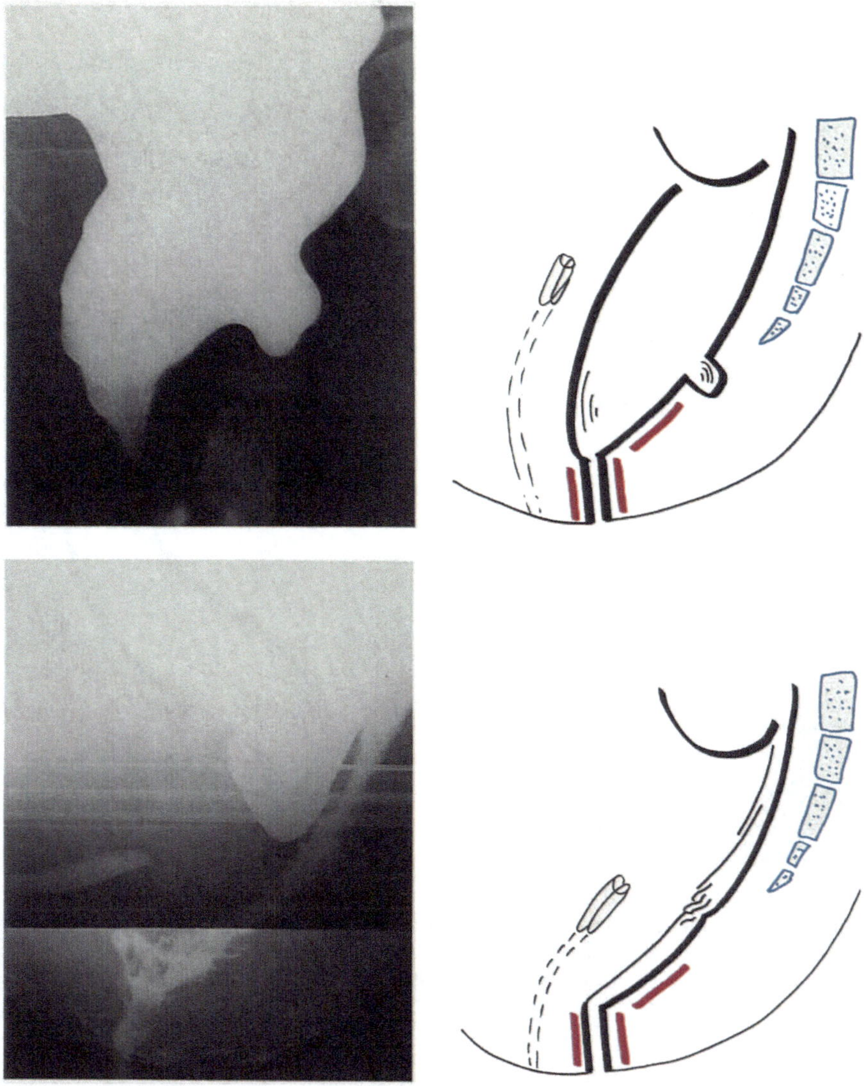

**Fig. 16.8.** *Above*: Small left lateral hernia, clearly distinguishable on lateral view. *Below*: During defaecation and contraction of levator ani muscle, hernia is pressed out and disappears

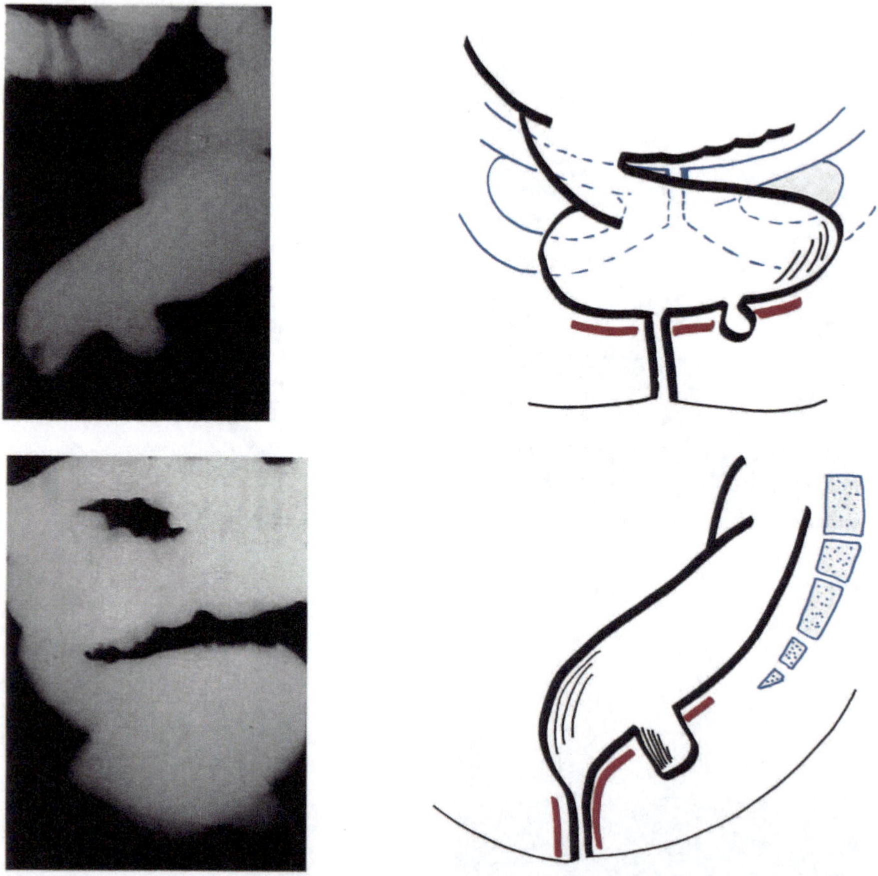

**Fig. 16.9.** *Above*: Rectal hernia in left lateral gap of levator ani muscle in a 51-year-old woman. Extent of sacculation is clearly seen on a.p. view. *Below*: Incomplete evacuation of rectum with rectocele on a.p. view; under defecation pressure and contraction of levator ani muscle, hernia does nor change in size

### *16.3.1.3 Small Hernias Enlarged by Evacuation*

Hernias with a diameter of 2–3 cm do not all remain unaltered on evacuation: some enlarge under intestinal pressure. A small diverticulum-like protrusion of the rectum becomes longer and larger and apparently penetrates further into the muscular pelvic floor (Fig. 16.10). In several patients we found incomplete evacuation associated with residues of stool in this kind of outpocketing.

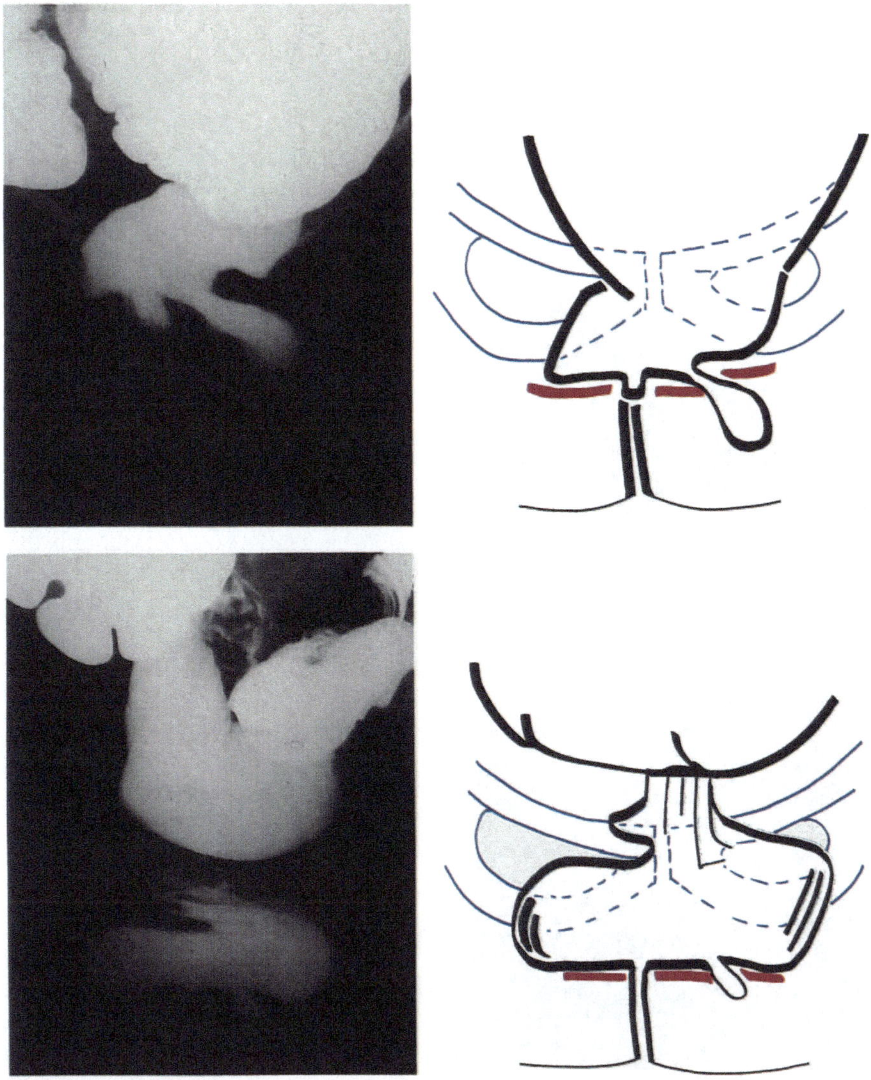

**Fig. 16.10.** *Above*: Left lateral hernia of about 2 cm in diameter in a 49-year-old woman. Up to this size there are no associated clinical findings at rest. *Below*: Under defecation pressure hernia enlarges and penetrates into the muscle layer. When faeces are pressed in this hernia the first sign of incomplete emptying appears

### *16.3.2 Medium-sized Hernias*

Hernias with a diameter of 3 cm or more regularly enlarge under defaecation pressure. Symptoms such as a feeling of incomplete evacuation is common. The size and location of these hernias may give the impression of a quite

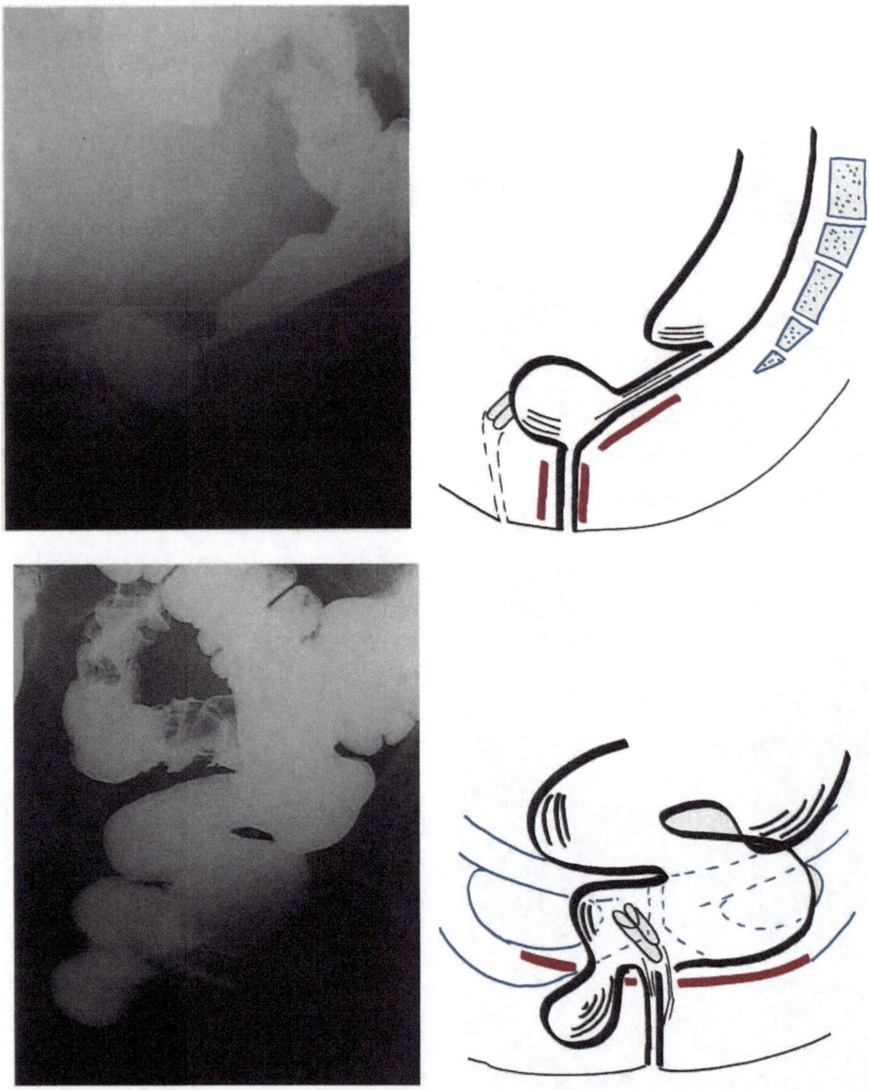

**Fig. 16.11.** *Above*: On lateral view this right lateral hernia in a 43-year-old woman may be confounded with rectocele. Uncommon for rectocele is a partly hidden tampon. *Below*: The a.p. view shows constant right lateral levator hernia. Hernia of levator muscle is seen in 6% of defaecograms

different diagnosis (Fig. 16.11). The x-ray film may demonstrate right lateral position of the hernia. Normally medium-sized hernias are invisible on double-contrast enema.

Figure 16.12 shows one of the rare left lateral hernias in male patients.

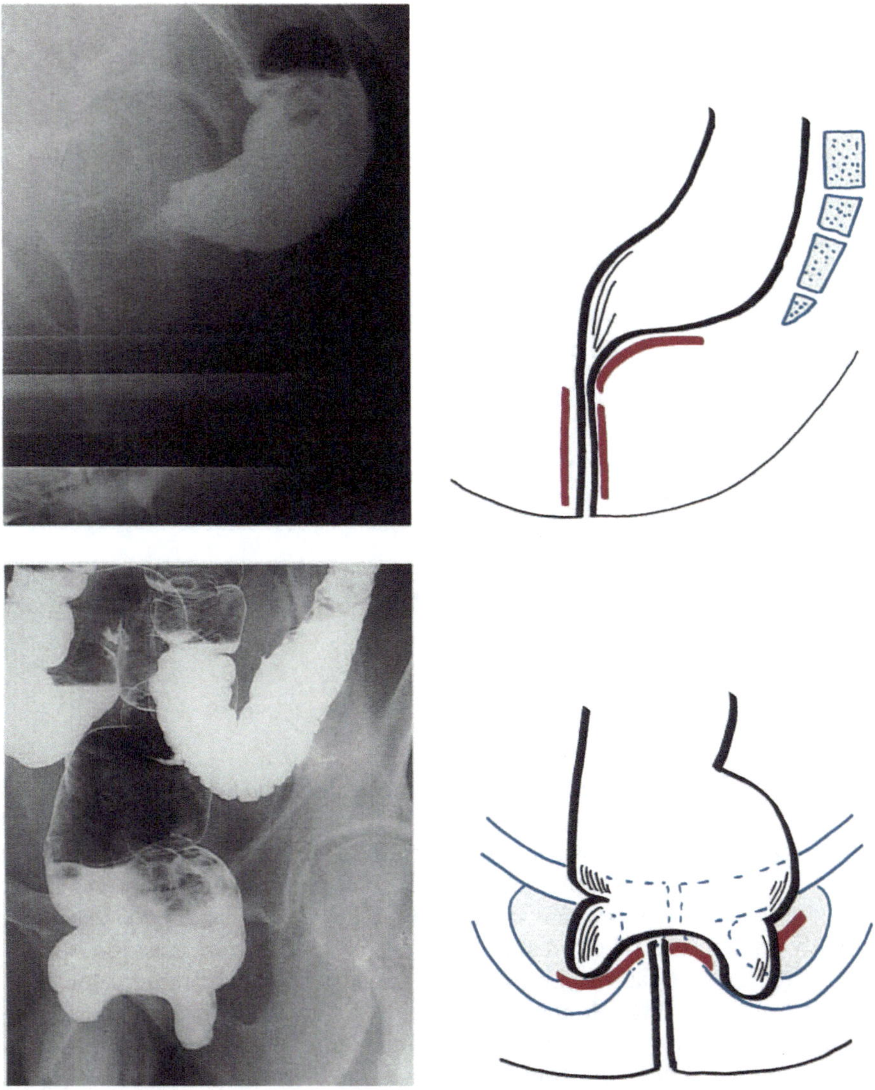

**Fig. 16.12.** *Above*: Levator hernia in a 49-year-old man, one of only three such hernias we have found in male patients. Lateral aspect of rectum appears normal. *Below*: The a.p. view shows sacculation on both sides, more extensive on the left than on the right. **Fig. 16.12** continues on p. 158

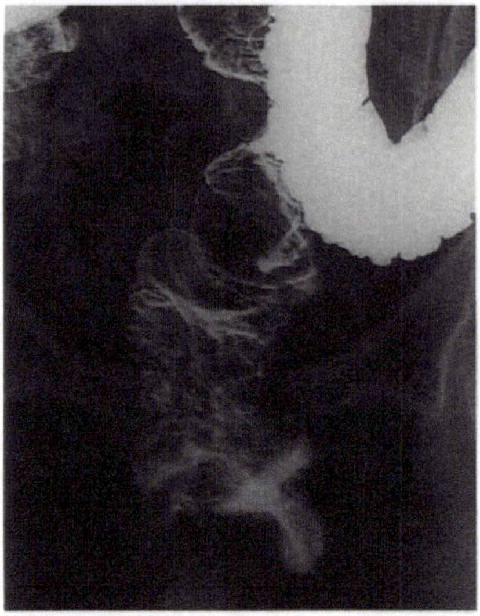

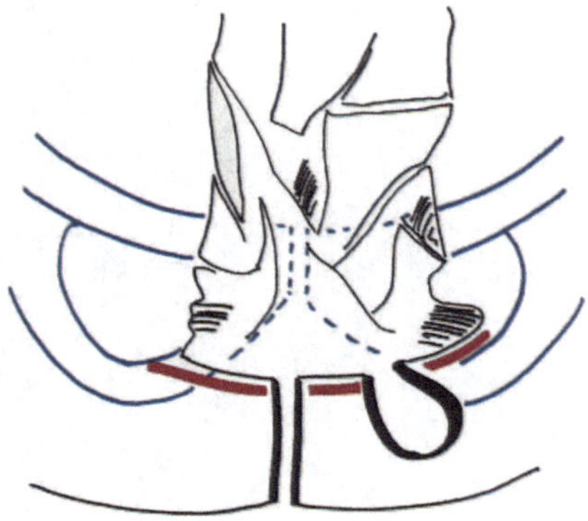

**Fig. 16.12** (*continued*). In the a.p. projection the evacuated rectum resembles a crumpled ribbon with a now enlarged left-sided sacculation

### *16.3.3 Large Hernias*

Large levator gap hernias are rare. In more than 2000 defaecographies we found only four of them. Every patient with this kind of hernia suffered from significant bowel evacuation problems from youth onward. They all needed to exert manual pressure on a certain point of their buttocks to be able to evacuate the rectum completely. The size of the hernia increases greatly under intestinal pressure. Figure 16.13 demonstrates the widening of the levator gap during straining. Large portions of the rectum can be pushed entirely through the gap. If only a lateral view is obtained the examiner sees evacuation but the remaining contrast medium in the hernia could simulate a filled portion of the rectum. A spastic pelvic floor syndrome [13] must therefore be excluded.

The double-contrast defaecography technique enables accurate assessment of the size and shape of larger hernias. In our experience this is mainly because of the different position of the patient during defaecography than on double-contrast enema examination or air instillation, when the out-pocketing is much smaller than in the sitting position. This is perhaps the reason why double-contrast enema and colonoscopy miss most hernias (Fig. 16.13).

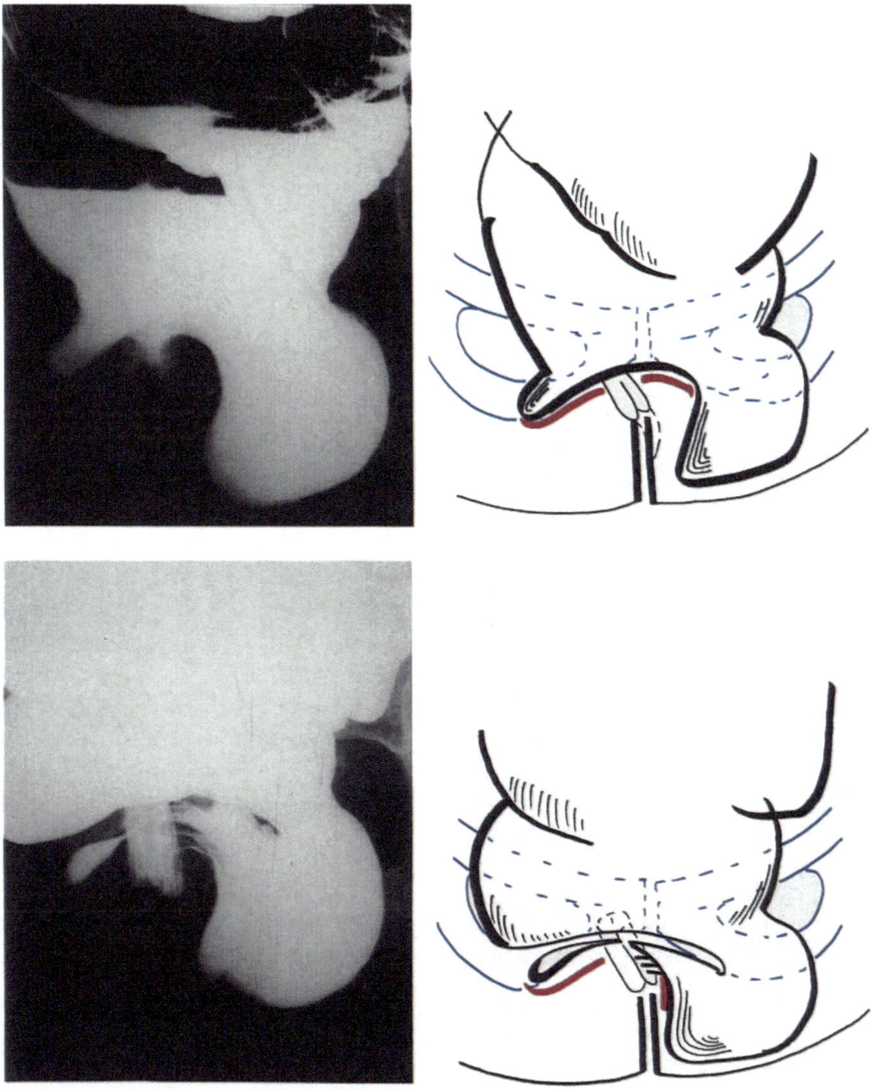

**Fig. 16.13.** *Above*: A 55-year-old woman had suffered her whole life from defaecation problems. Complete evacuation was only possible if she pressed a certain point on her left buttock. The drawing explains the left lateral hernia on the a.p. view *Below*: On defaecation a rectal loop is pressed into the large levator muscle gap. Entrance of anal canal is much higher than content of hernia. Evacuation is only possible when stool is lifted above anal canal level by described manoeuvre. **Fig. 16.13** continues on p. 160

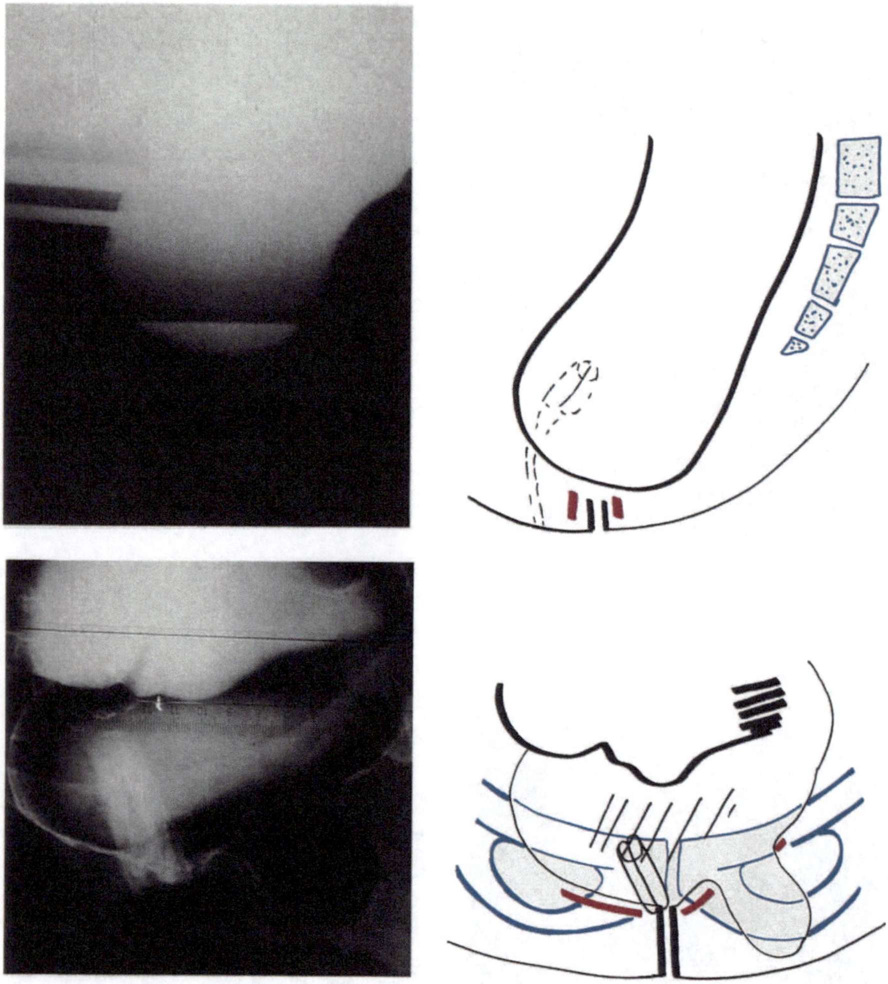

**Fig. 16.13** (*continued*). *Above*: Lateral view of evacuated rectum. Mass of remaining rectal content may give impression of spastic pelvic floor. *Below*: On double-contrast enema inflated air shows left lateral hernia with patient in prone position. Only large hernias are visible on double-contrast enema

## 16.4 Non-ventral Bending, Folding or Outpocketing of the Rectum

Rectoceles and levator gap hernias arise from muscular or connective tissue weakness. The description of dorsal, lateral and zigzag-shaped outpocketings that now follows is mainly based upon evaluation of a.p. radiographs and rotating fluoroscopy. The recent literature on defaecography seems to contain no thoroughgoing evaluation of a.p. views; our own findings are presented below.

Bending, folding or outpocketing of the rectum can be considered as the result of some special features of rectal anatomy. As we could show in Chap. 3, intestinal pressure acts according to a parallelogram of forces in a craniocandal and in a more ventrodorsal way. This should in some way shorten the rectum along a longitudinal axis and diminish the ventrodorsal diameter.

On the other hand, there are muscular fibers in is the rectum wall itself, which form a helix of about 54° [19]. When emptied, muscular fibers contract and provoke mucosal folds at three points known as Houston I, II and III. These mucosal folds may vary individually, just as the length of the anal canal, the insertion of the peritoneum or the form of the os coccygis vary. It may also be important how far lateral excursion and extension of the rectum in the pelvis are possible.

Thus, the interaction of traction, pressure and shearing forces can displace the rectum from its normal straight alignment. The basic analysis of defaecograms is described in Chap. 6. Additional information on non-ventral bends, folds and outpocketings can be obtained in the a.p. projection. This view should be taken with the patient sitting rather than standing. Our comparative study has shown that if the findings are questionable in the lateral projection an a.p. view with the standing patient pressing against his sphincters can provide clarity.

### *16.4.1 Rectal Prolapse and Intussusception: Three-Dimensional Analysis*

Many authors agree that the first sign of that rectal prolapse is intussusception [2, 3, 6, 8, 9, 11, 15, 17]. Mahieu et al. and Ekberg et al. showed that rectal prolapse begins with the onset of intussusception at the upper rim of the anal canal or higher in the rectum, describing it as the ring pocket sign [7] or the "en champignon" aspect [16]. We find this clear and reproducible phenomenon in our patients too (Fig. 16.14), at the upper rim of the anal canal. Smooth rectal mucosa can be found in the lumen of the canal. Many authors report this phenomenon of rectal prolapse with invagination [5, 10, 12, 15]. In many cases, apparent rectal intussusception on lateral proctography, with or without complete evacuation of the rectum, is revealed on an a.p. view to be not only an anterior mucosal prolapse but also a zigzag folding resembling a concertina. There is no evidence in such patients for

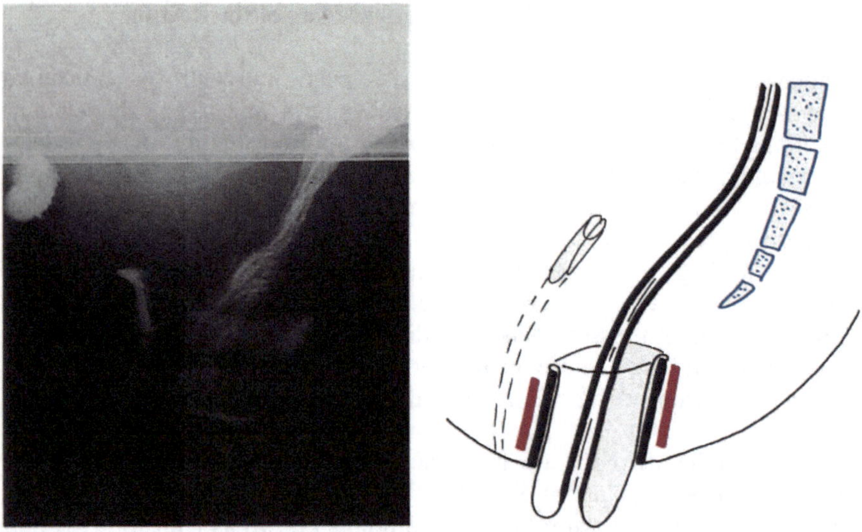

**Fig. 16.14.** Rectal intussusception and prolapse through anal canal. Circular onset on smooth mucosal surface (ring pocket sign). No additional folds are seen

the existence of intussusception above the anal canal or in the anal canal itself. Bends and folds vary intraindividually and become deeper with forced straining. A bend or fold that is deeply unpressed into the pelvic floor overlies this deviated anal canal in the lateral projection so that it seems to disappear. We observed in 200 defaecograms in a.p. projection or with fluoroscopy that bends vary in shape when the patient strains repeatedly. In 93% of patients we found a zigzag bending or folding sometimes the anal canal seems to disappear in lateral view at the bottom of a "funnel-like intussusception". In a.p. view, this can be explained by a deviation to the left or to the right.
Three states that may lead to misdiagnosis of intussusception are (1) funnel-like deformation of the anal canal in the lateral projection, (2) invagination-like deformation of the midrectum in the lateral projection and (3) multilocular deformation of the rectum with retention of barium.

### *16.4.2.1 Funnel-Like Deformation of the Anal Canal*

Figure 16.15 (above) shows, in the lateral projection, a funnel-like configuration of preanal mucosal folds. Parts of a "ring pocket" can be distinguished, and the rectal contour enters the funnel. On an a.p. view (Fig. 16.15 below) the anal canal is visible. The funnel-like folds emerge as a rectal bend to the right and a rectal fold to the left.

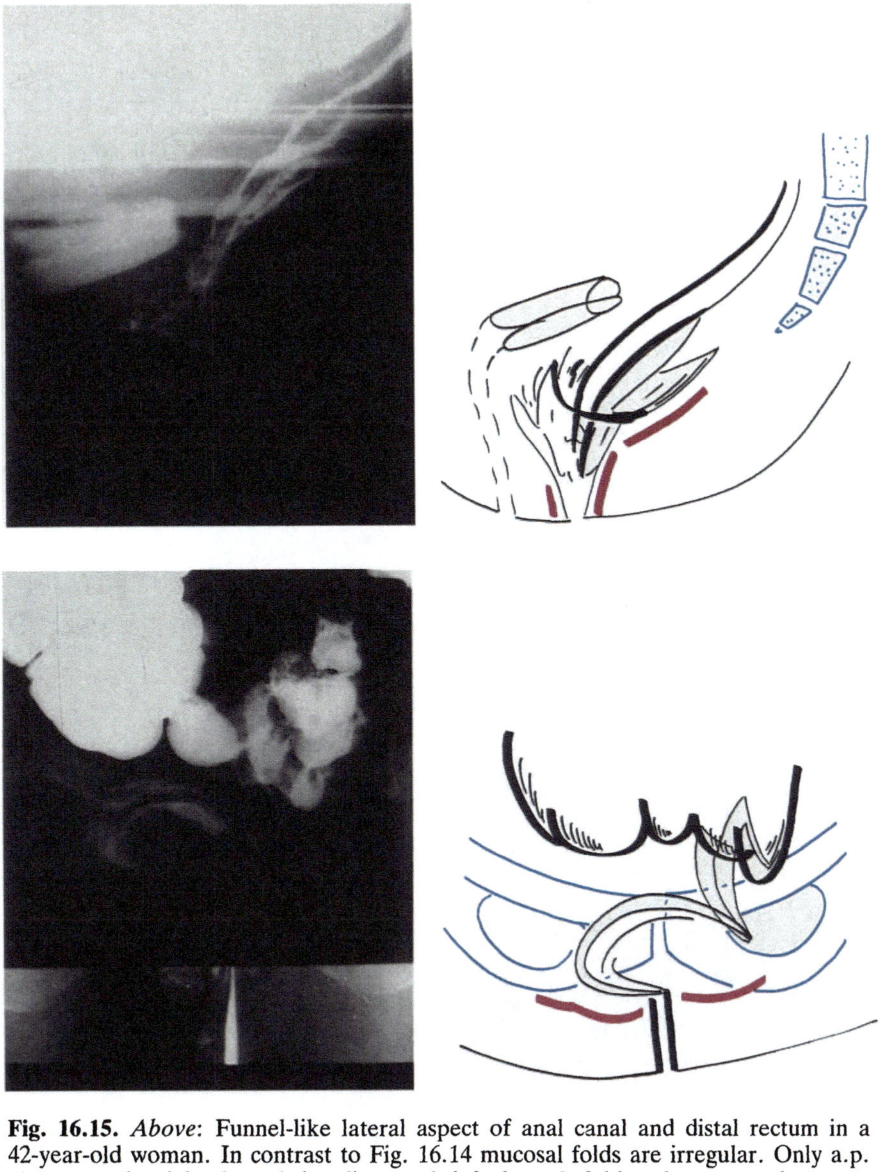

**Fig. 16.15.** *Above*: Funnel-like lateral aspect of anal canal and distal rectum in a 42-year-old woman. In contrast to Fig. 16.14 mucosal folds are irregular. Only a.p. view reveals right lateral bending and left lateral folds of evacuated rectum resembling a concertina. Folds vary with intestinal pressure

### *16.4.2.2 Invagination-Like Deformation of Midrectum*

Figure 16.6 (above) shows, in the lateral projection, a mid-rectal invagination above a not completely opacified "rectocele" over an inclined anal canal. On the a.p. view (Fig. 16.16 below) the mostly evacuated rectum

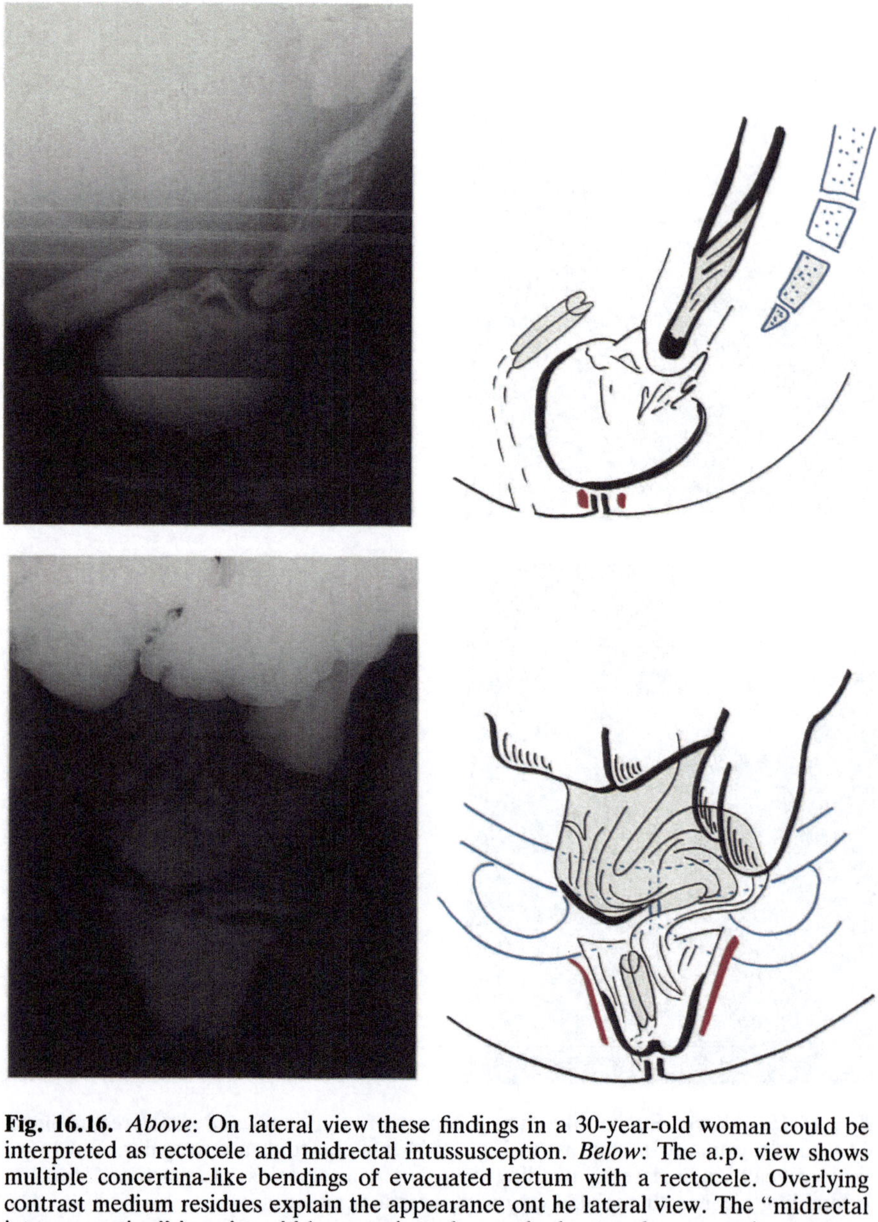

**Fig. 16.16.** *Above*: On lateral view these findings in a 30-year-old woman could be interpreted as rectocele and midrectal intussusception. *Below*: The a.p. view shows multiple concertina-like bendings of evacuated rectum with a rectocele. Overlying contrast medium residues explain the appearance ont he lateral view. The "midrectal intussusception" is a sigmoid loop projected over the bent and evacuated rectum

zigzags from right to left and back. One bend to the right contains a residue of barium, and this is superimposed on an evacuated part of rectum on the lateral view.

#### *16.4.2.3 Multilocular Deformation of Rectum with Retention of Barium*

Barium retention in the rectum often gives the patient the feeling of incomplete evacuation. On a lateral view (Fig. 16.17 above) multilocular retentions are seen. Repeated efforts at evacuation do not alter these trapped, barium-filled pockets. On the a.p. view (Fig. 16.17 below) multiple concertina-like bends of the rectum explain the appearance on the lateral view. When the patient strains strongly, the folds fill with barium or stool while adjacent sections of the rectum are squeezed. The last fold (to the right!) can be pressed into the pelvic floor so that the anal canal is invisible on the lateral view.

## 16.5 Dorsal Outpocketings

We found dorsal outpocketings in 3% of the patients we examined. Evacuation is incomplete. Pathophysiology of this type of outpocketing can be clarified only by means of examination methods other than defaecography (Fig. 16.18).

## 16.6 Rare and Combined Outpocketings

One unusual type of hernia, which we have observed in only one patient, is a hernia lateral to or within the anococcygeal ligament (Fig. 16.19). Various combinations of different subtypes of rectal outpocketings have been observed. In our experience a combination of rectocele and concertina-like bends is not infrequent.

In folds of the rectum tension and compression of the rectal mucosa can presumably induce defects of the mucosal surface resembling superficial ulcerative scars in double-contrast enema. Spotted contrast medium patterns can occasionally be observed 24 h after forced defaection for barium enema (Fig. 16.20). This rare lesion has not yet been clearly interpreted in the literature [1].

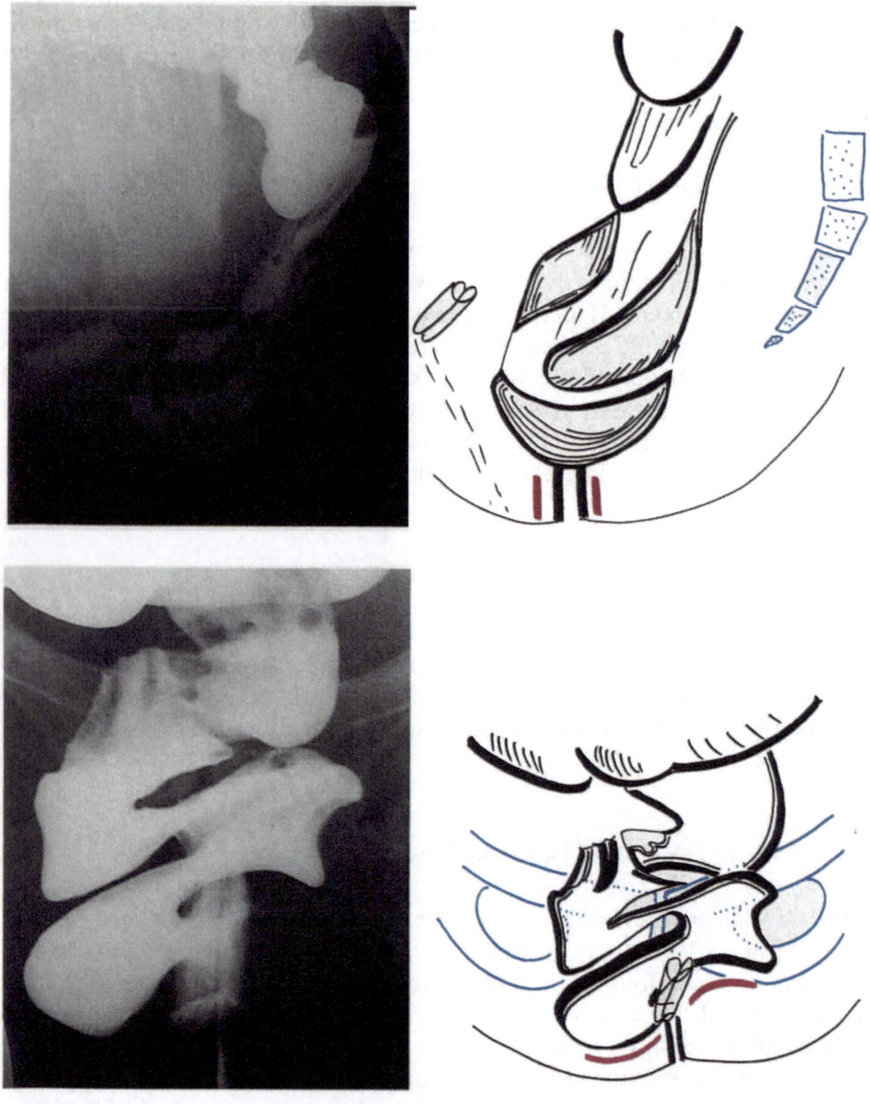

**Fig. 16.17.** *Above*: In a 63-year-old woman, irregularly shaped contrast residues gave an impression of incomplete evacuation. *Below*: The a.p. view shows distribution of contrast residues in right and left lateral bends and pockets in a concertina-like rectum

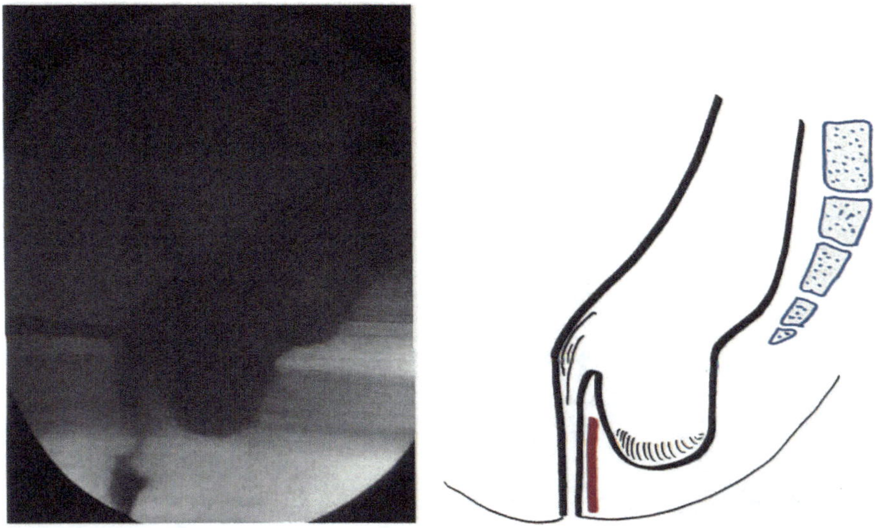

**Fig. 16.18.** In very rare cases, as in this 52-year-old woman, the anal canal is pushed forward, making room for a dorsal outpocketing where normally the pubococcygeal muscle or ligament is found

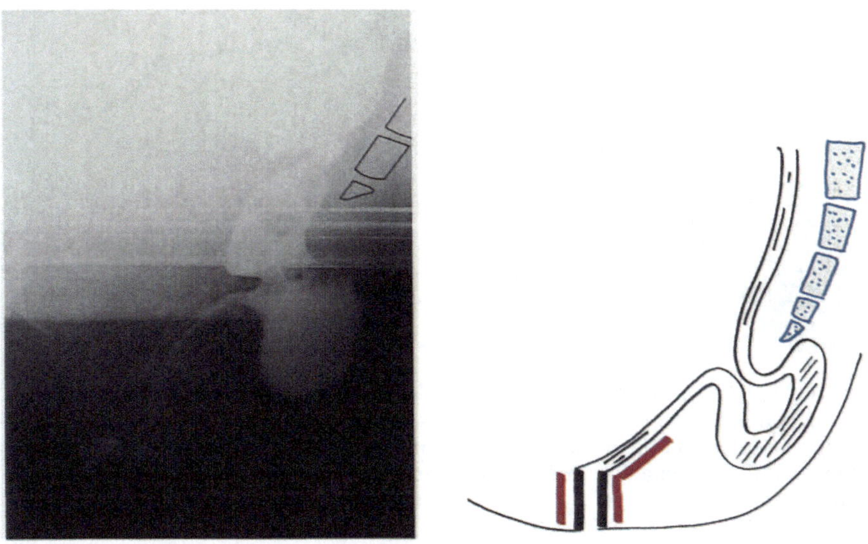

**Fig. 16.19.** Dorsal outpocketing in form of midline hernia immediately below coccygeal bone

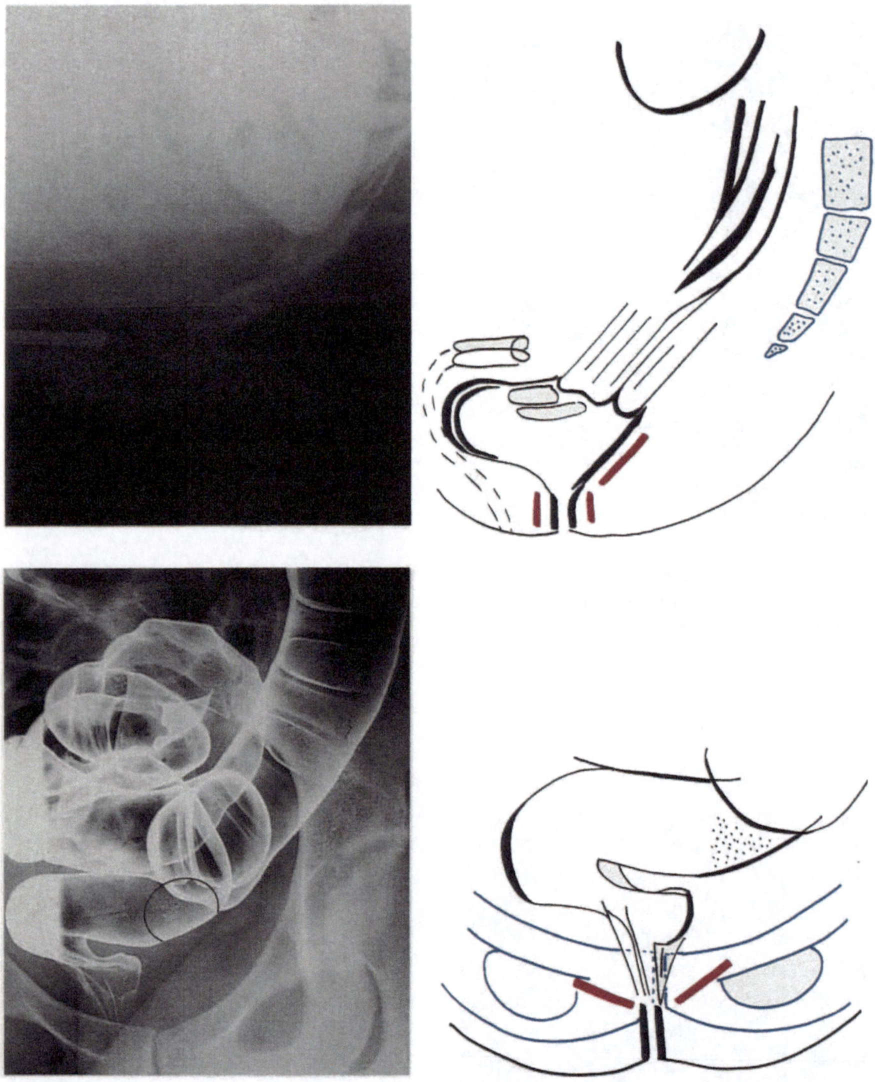

Fig. 16.20. *Above*: Rectocele and rectal folds in a 35-year-old woman. *Below*: When defaecation before double-contrast enema is strong enough and patient presses long enough on folds and bends of rectum, superficial barium dots like scars are seen on double contrast enema 24 h later, on the same side as a simple rectal ulcer seen on colonoscopy

## 16.7 Conclusion

Modification of the functional defaecography examination technique to include anteroposterior views (x-ray and fluoroscopy) allows distinction between solitary, multiple and multilocular subtypes of rectal outpocketings.

Defaecography is used to show rectal hernias and to observe how they deform under intestinal pressure.
The anteroposterior projection renders defaecography able to localize concertina-like bends and folds, especially if they do not evacuate completely. In many cases structures adjoining these outpocketings can be identified using contrast medium. Together with a history of diagnosis and clinical symptoms, functional defaecography makes therapeutic procedures more specific and successful.

## References


1. Altaras J (1982) Radiologischer Atlas: Colon und Rectum. Urban and Schwarzenberg, Munich
2. Bartram CI, Turnball GK, Lennard-Jones JE (1988) Evacuation proctography: an investigation of rectal expulsion in 20 subjects without defecatory disturbance. Gastrointest Radiol 13:72–80
3. Berman IR, Harris MF, Leggett IT (1987) Rectal reservoir reduction procedures for internal rectal prolapse. Dis Colon Rectum
4. Berretta O, Chaussade S, Coquet M, Couturier D, Bonnin A, Guerre J (1990) Technique simplifiée de défecographie. Description et résultats. Presse Med 19(33)
5. Choi DL, Ekberg O (1988) Functional analysis of anorectal junction: defecography. ROFO 148:50–53
6. Devadhar DSC (1964) New thoughts on the mechanism and treatment of rectal procidentia. J Int Coll Surg 42:672–681
7. Ekberg O, Nylander G, Fork FT (1985) Defecography. Radiology 155:45–48
8. Felt-Bersma RJF, Luth WJ, Janssen JJWM, Meuwissen SGM (1990) Defecography in patients with anorectal disorders. Dis Colon Rectum
9. Goei R, Baeten C (1990) Rectal intussusception and rectal prolapse: detection and postoperative evaluation with defecography. Radiology 174:124–126
10. Goei R, Baeten C, Arends JW (1988) Solitary rectal ulcer syndrome: findings at barium enema study and defecography. Radiology 168:303–306
11. Kelly-Mickus G (1989) Defecography: a new technique for the study of disorders of defecation. Radiography Today 55
12. Kuijpers JHC, de Morree H (1988) Toward a selection of the most appropriate procedure in the treatment of complete rectal prolapse. Dis Colon Rectum
13. Kuijpers HC, Bleijenberg G (1985) The spastic pelvic floor syndrome. Dis Colon Rectum
14. Mahieu PHG (1990) Défécographie, explorations fonctionelles. Ann Gastroénterol Hepatol 26(4):161–165
15. Mahieu P, Pringot J, Bodart P (1984) Defecography: II. contribution to the diagnosis of defecation disorders. Gastrointest Radiol 9:253–261
16. Mahieu P, Pringot J, Vanheuverzwijn R, Goncette L (1981) Les prolapsus du rectum. Acta Gastroenterol Belg, 44: Vol XLIV
17. Shorvon PJ, McHugh S, Diamant NE, Somers S (1989) Defecography in normal volunteers: results and implications. Gut 30:1737–1749
18. Waldeyer A (1967) Anatomie des Menschen. De Gruyter, Berlin
19. Lierse W (1984) Becken. In: von Lanz T, Wachsmuth R (eds) Praktische Anatomie, Vol 2 Teil 8A, Springer, Berlin Heidelberg New York

# 17 Enterocele

R. Hauck

## 17.1 Introduction

Enteroceles are visualised by defaecography and have frequently been described, mostly in the form of case reports [2, 4–6, 12, 19, 25, 26]. Gynaecologists are often confronted by the consequences of enteroceles [1, 3, 7, 10, 11, 13, 15, 16, 18, 20–24, 27–30]. During routine gynaecological examinations, the frequency of enterocele is about 2%–3% [17]. However, in patients requiring major gynaecological procedures, Ranney [22] noted an incidence of 18.1%.

Of 2000 patients with defaecation disorders investigated by us, 17.4% suffered from enteroceles. Opening of the pouch of Douglas and interposition of colon/small intestine or other tissue represents a hernia with

- Hernial aperture
- Hernial sac
- Hernial contents

Relevant questions are:

- How can defaecography contribute to the recognition of such hernias?
- To what extent does defaecography visualise the effects of larger hernias on adjacent organs?
- How do enteroceles differ after hysterectomy?

## 17.2 Radiological Technique

The defaecographic technique should follow the guidelines set out in Sect. 5.1. Localisation of the uterus in patients with an intra-uterine contraceptive device (IUD) may be helpful. In our experience the position of a contrast-soaked tampon within the vagina and of an IUD remains constant at rest and under defaecation pressure; this means that if the uterus moves away from the rectum, the tampon does too (e.g. when the pouch of Douglas is open).

## 17.3 Defaecographic Criteria Enteria of Hernias

The *hernialaperture* consists of or is limited by:

- The vagina ventrally
- The rectum dorsally
- The uterosacral ligaments laterally

Both the vagina and the rectum are contrasted and radiopaque in defaecography, while the uterosacral ligaments are not. In several patients with small hernias we found an impression of the sigmoid colon at the point of intersection between the uterosacral ligaments and this part of the herniated colon. The shape of unpressed sigma may be that of a bow [Figs. 17.1, 17.2] or of a finger [Figs. 17.3, 17.4]. From a radiological point of view the insertion of uterosacral ligaments on the uterus may be localized if:

- The center of uterus is marked by IUD or
- The vaginal vault is marked by contrast soaked tampon and
- The sigmoid colon typically pressed into the pouch of Douglas.

Because of the tight and normally invariable relation between uterus and vaginal vault, the tampon-marked vagina alone gives us localisation of ligaments. Even after hysterectomy, the relationship between ligaments and tampon remains intact because ligaments are commonly sutured with vaginal stump.

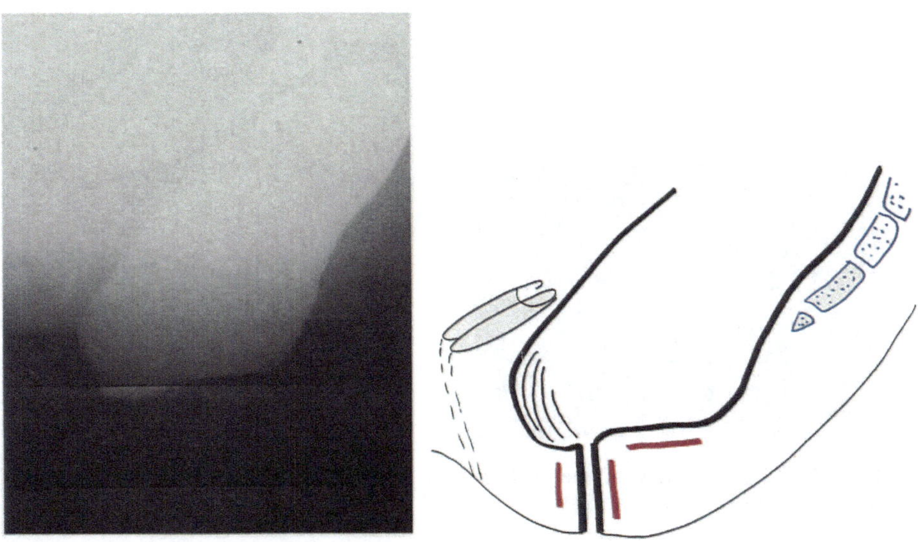

**Fig. 17.1.** Lateral view of the rectum in a 45-year-old patient with an IUD; no pathological sign is seen at rest. For key to colours, see p. 26

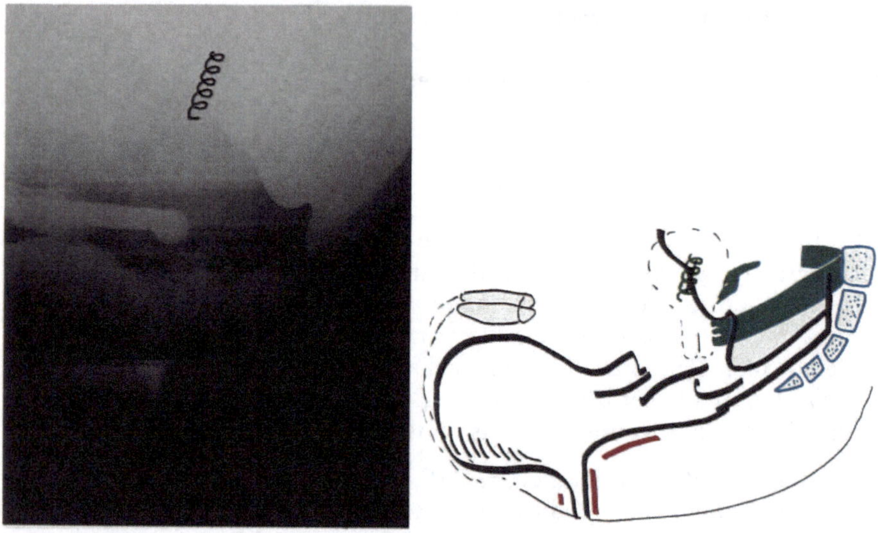

**Fig. 17.2.** Same patient as in Fig. 17.1. At defaecation part of the sigmoid colon squeezes between the uterosacral ligaments. A step-like impression of the ventral part of the sigmoid colon is caused by the uterus and the uterosacral ligaments. These hold back the uterus like reins

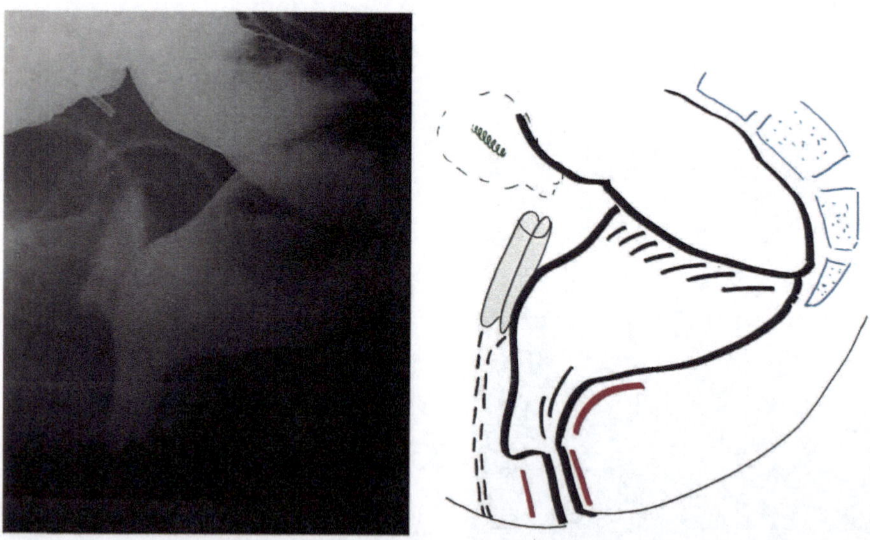

**Fig. 17.3.** Lateral view of the rectum in a 47-year-old patient with an IUD; no pathological sign is seen at rest

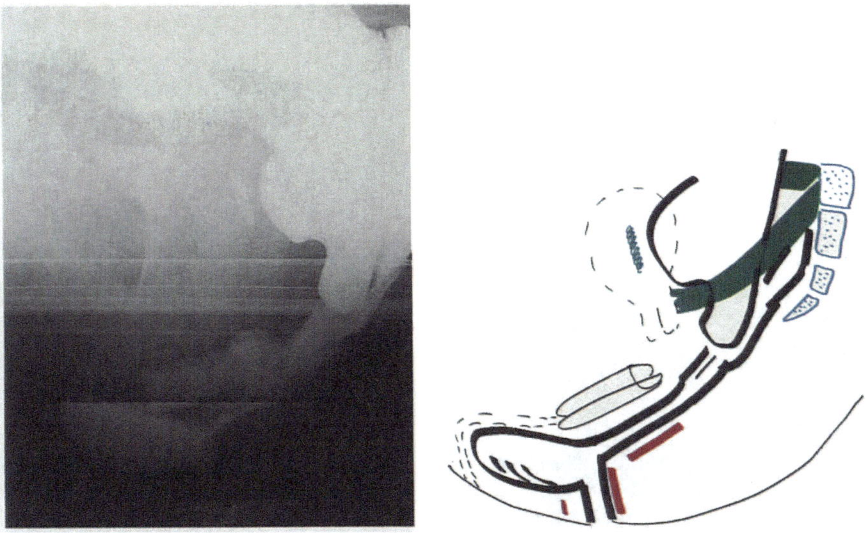

**Fig. 17.4.** Same patient as in Fig. 17.3. At defaecation a tiny, finger-like portion of the sigmoid colon enters the pouch of Douglas, representing the onset of enterocele. The difference between Figs. 17.4 and 17.2 lies in the dorsal shape of impressed sigmoid colon. A step-like alteration in the anterior wall of sigmoid colon is typical for the onset of enteroceles

**Table 17.1.** Contents of the hernia in 348 patients with enterocele, as revealed by defaecography

| | |
|---|---|
| Colon | 39.0% |
| Small intestine | 31.7% |
| Small intestine and colon combined | 2.4% |
| Content identified | 73.1% |
| Content unidentified | 26.9% |

If we know consequently the insertion point of ligaments, we can draw a line to the onset of ligaments on the 4th sacral vertebra and thus have that position on our x-ray exposure.

In this way we can define hernial aperture by the constructed course of ligaments and the radiolucent parts of the vaginal vault and the rectum.

The *hernial sac* consists of peritoneum and is non-radiolucent in enteroceles. There is an "empty halo" between contrasted rectum in the pouch of Douglas and vaginal tissue.

The *contents of the hernia* can be distinguished by defaecography (Table 17.1):

- Interposition of colon can be recognised owing to the contrast medium (Figs. 17.5, 17.6)

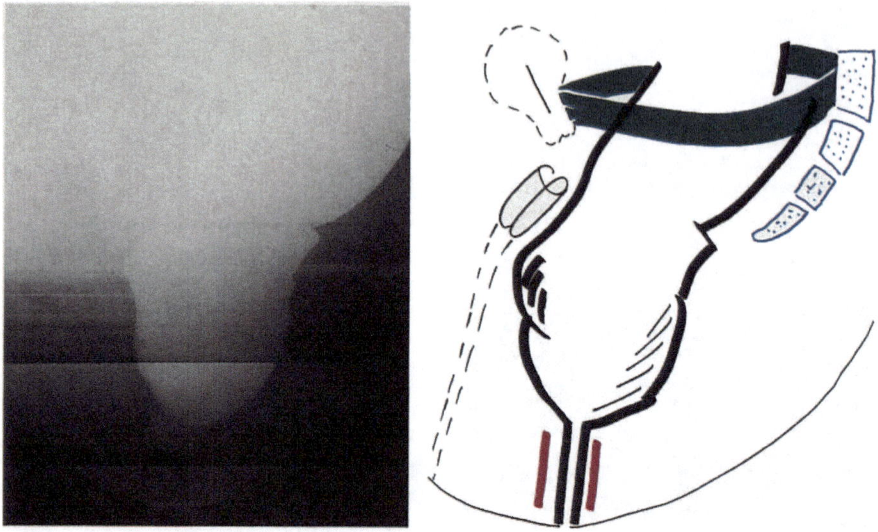

**Fig. 17.5.** Lateral view of the rectum at rest in a 52-year-old patient with a subjective feeling of incomplete evacuation. Normal finding

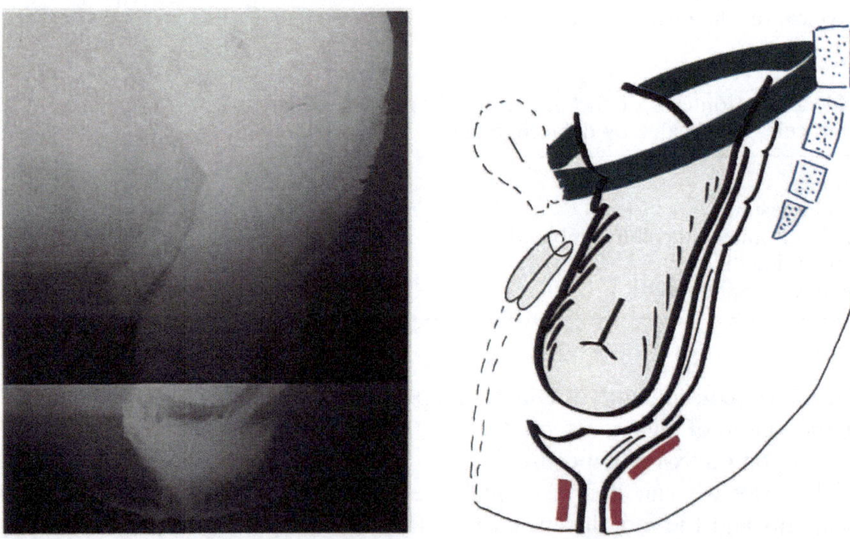

**Fig. 17.6.** Same patient as in Fig. 17.5. At defaecation there is formation of enterocele. Content of hernia: sigmoid colon

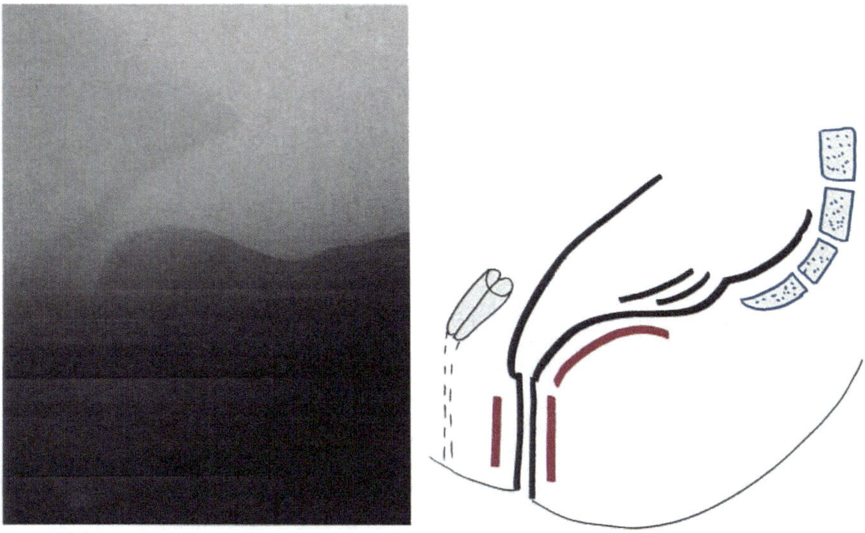

**Fig. 17.7.** Lateral view of the rectum at rest in a 39-year-old patient with a feeling of incomplete evacuation. Normal finding

- Interposition of small intestine is evident owing to the contrast medium (Figs. 17.7, 17.8) or air bubbles or enteric
- origin (Figs. 17.9, 17.10)
- Interposition of both the colon and small intestine is less frequent (Figs. 17.11, 17.12).

In 26.9% of our patients with enteroceles, there was an interposition of radiologically homogeneous tissue. Because of complete colonic opacification, we interpreted this homogeneous mass either as air-free small intestine or as other radiologically unidentifiable tissue. [26]

## 17.4 Defaecographic Appearance of Larger Enteroceles

Under conditions of intestinal pressure for defaecation and in a sitting position, two forms of larger enteroceles in contact with adjacent organic structures may be observed.

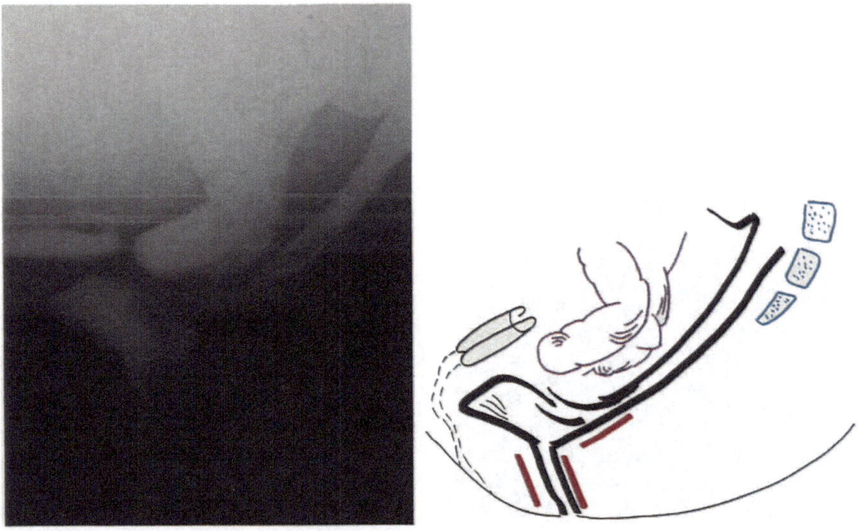

**Fig. 17.8.** Same patient as in Fig. 17.7. At defaecation, barium-contrasted small intestine enters the hernial sac. The rectocele is almost completely evacuated by the pressure of the enterocele

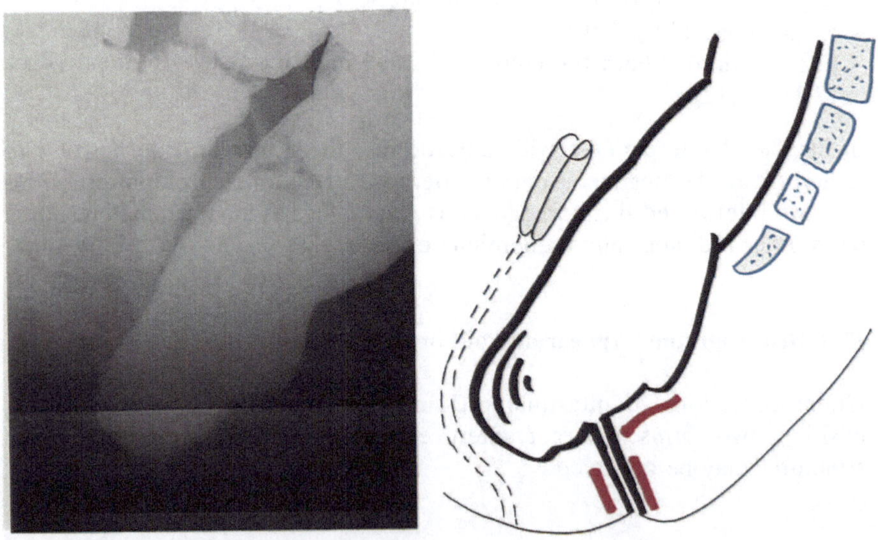

**Fig. 17.9.** Lateral view of the rectum. At rest outpocketing of a rectocele is clearly seen in this 47 year old patient

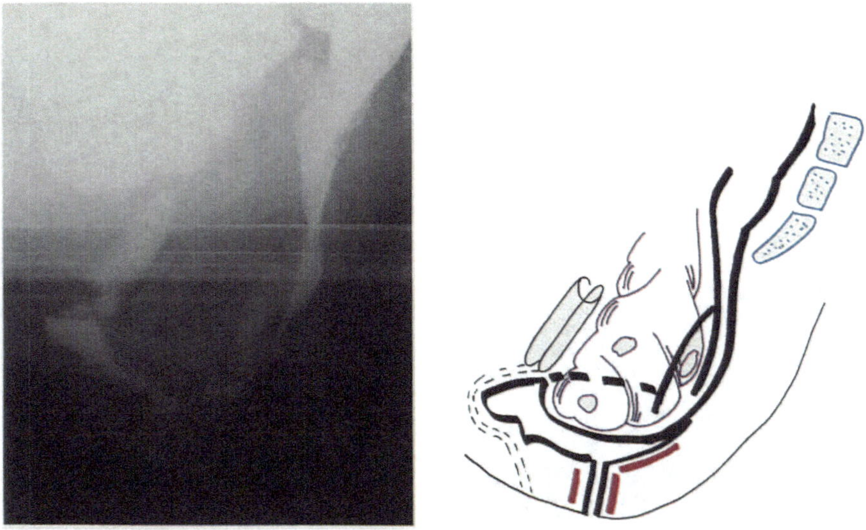

**Fig. 17.10.** Same patient as in Fig. 17.9. Air bubbles are present between the vagina and the empty rectum. The rectal out-pocketing is enlarged under intestinal pressure

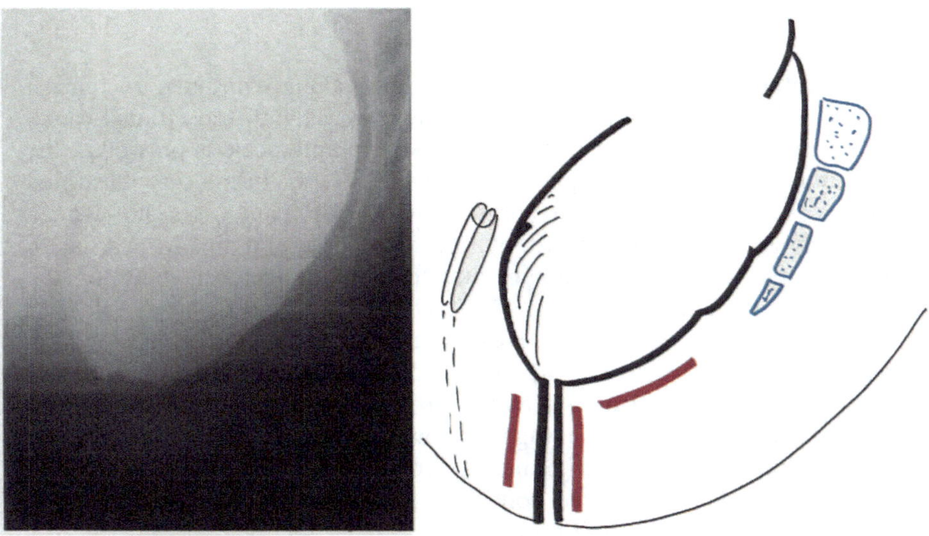

**Fig. 17.11.** Lateral view of rectum. A long anal canal is present, but no pathological sign is evident at rest

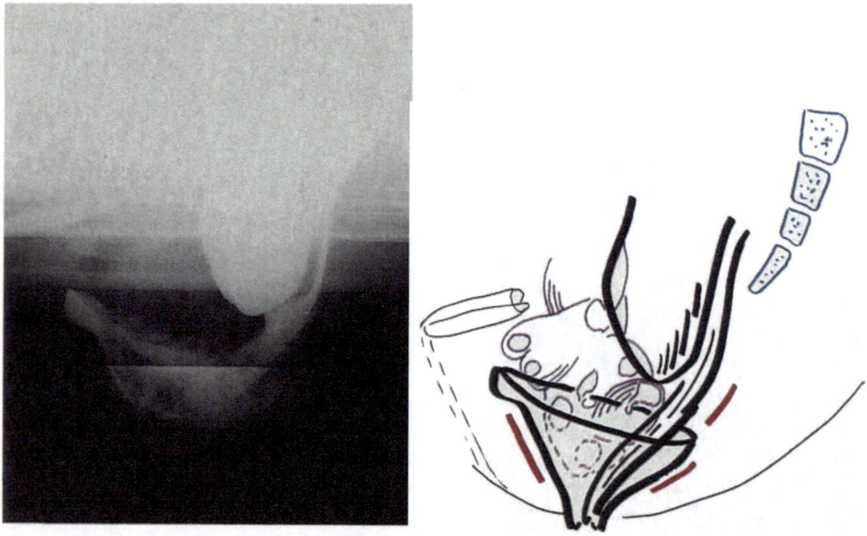

**Fig. 17.12.** Same 40-year-old patient as in Fig. 17.11. A large enterocele is seen, of which the hernial sac is filled by barium-contrasted sigmoid colon and air bubbles from the small intestine. The distended funnel-like anal canal indicates the initial stages of weakening of the muscular pelvic floor and the onset of anal prolapse

### *17.4.1 Vaginal Prolapse*

If an enterocele is viewed on its way down along evacuated rectum, it follows the perineal curve and slips easily over a tightly closed anal canal. When pressure lasts for a sufficient period, the enterocele is pressed in the direction of the introitus vaginae (Figs. 17.13, 17.14). In the case illustrated in Figs. 17.13 and 17.14 no rectocele is evident; in many cases, however, a rectocele is pushed downward by the enterocele and finally evacuated. Radiographs then show a tongue-like remnant of rectocele between the vagina and the enterocele (Figs. 17.15, 17.16).
In our experience with voluminous enteroceles, no major prolapse of the vagina could be diagnosed in patients under-going defaecography; even if there was evidence of such a prolapse when the patients were standing. The only major prolapse of the vagina known to us was cited in a personal communication from Marti (Geneva). Probably the sitting position adopted in the x-ray device and the contrast-soaked foreign body in the vagina hamper the enterocele from prolapsing.

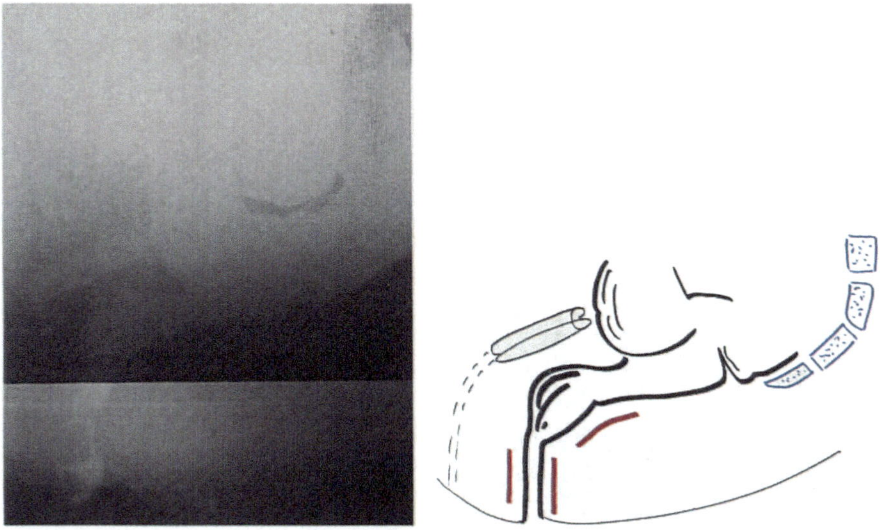

**Fig. 17.13.** Lateral view of rectum in a 63-year-old patient; deep sigmoid loop

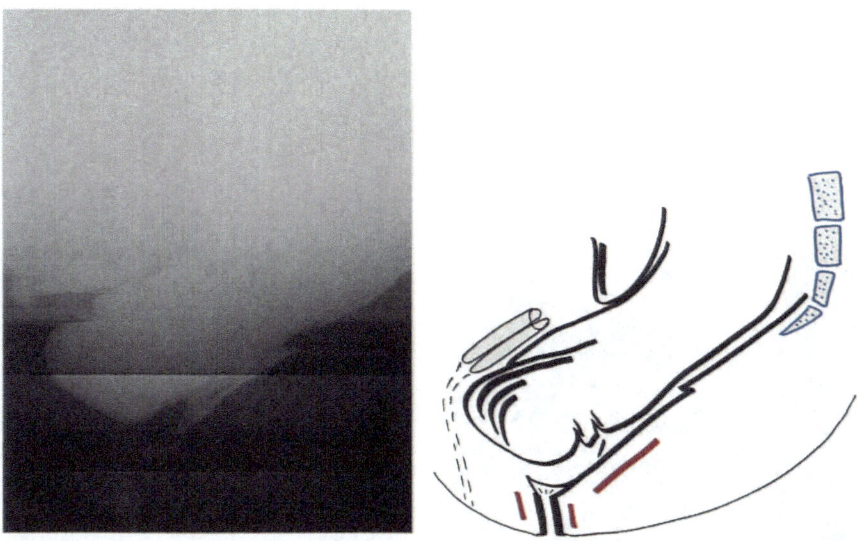

**Fig. 17.14.** Same patient as in Fig. 17.13. Enterocele contains sigmoid colon. The muscular pelvic floor is intact, so the enterocele has a tendency to form a vaginal prolapse

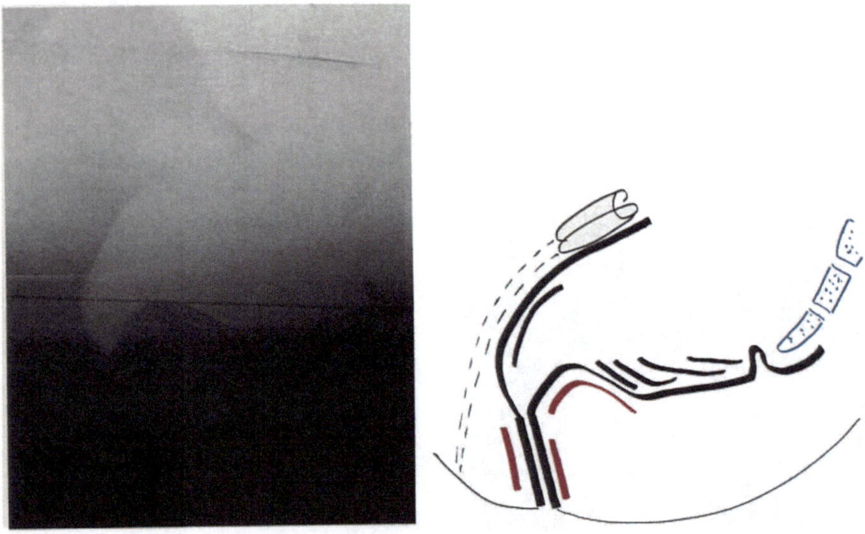

**Fig. 17.15.** Lateral view of the rectum in a 49-year-old patient. At rest impression of the puborectal sling is seen

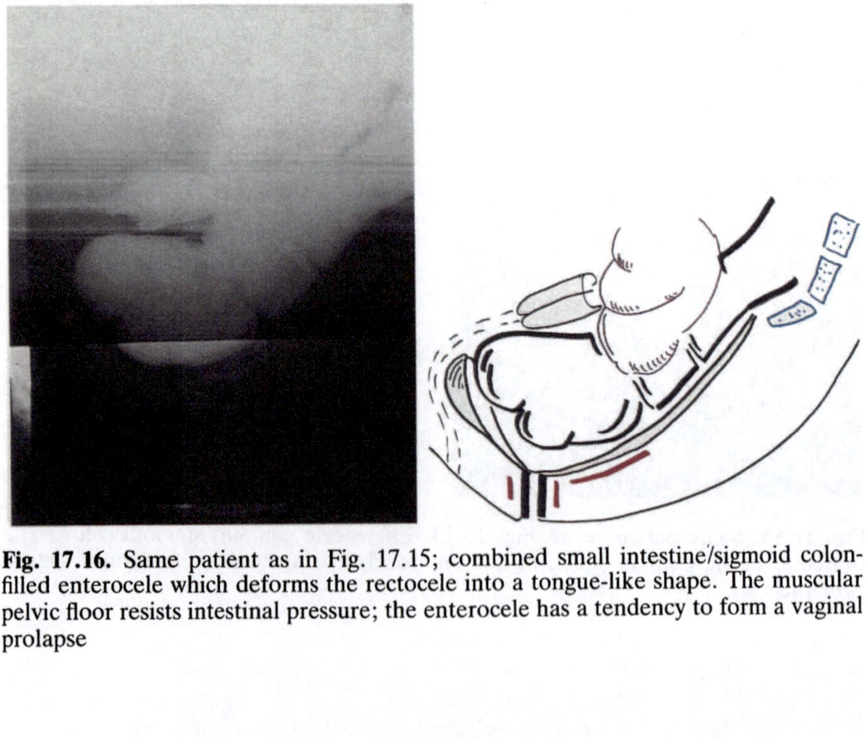

**Fig. 17.16.** Same patient as in Fig. 17.15; combined small intestine/sigmoid colon-filled enterocele which deforms the rectocele into a tongue-like shape. The muscular pelvic floor resists intestinal pressure; the enterocele has a tendency to form a vaginal prolapse

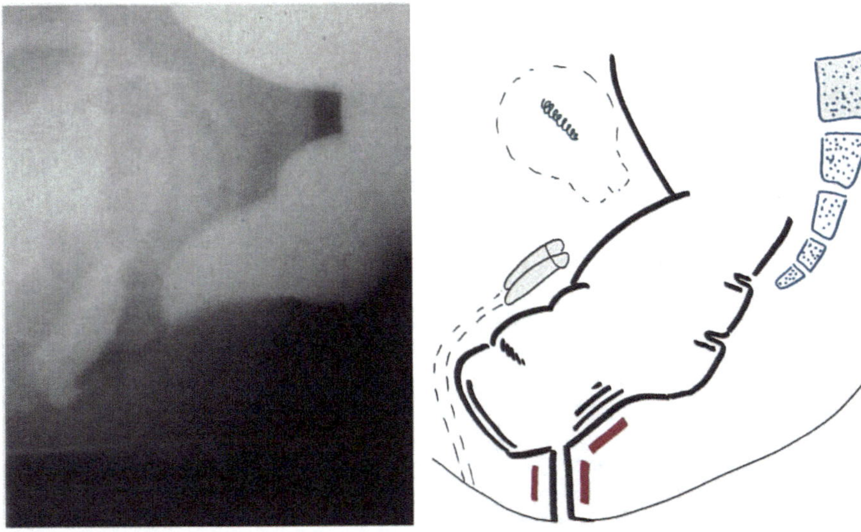

**Fig. 17.17.** Lateral view of the rectum at rest in a 39-year-old patient with an IUD

### *17.4.2 Anal/Rectal Prolapse*

A second form of larger enteroceles affects the muscular pelvic floor. If the anal canal is not so tightly closed, the enterocele interposes between the more circular muscles around the anal canal, thereby distending it; this may produce a more funnel-like shape (Figs. 17.12, 17.17, 17.18). Alternatively, the enterocele sits like an egg in an egg cup (Figs. 17.19, 17.20). Distension may vary. In cases of extreme weakening of the pelvic floor, the superior rectal wall is pressed out through the anal canal and appears as a prolapse with a "doubled" anal canal. Remaining rectocele is clearly seen. Finally all the anal canal may be everted, forming a complete rectal prolapse containing enterocele (Figs. 17.21, 17.22).

## 17.5 Special Observations

### *17.5.1 Very Small Enteroceles*

In several cases we saw a distance of 2–3 cm between contrast-soaked tampon and evacuated rectum. This distance was not large enough to distinguish between e.g. thickened rectal wall and onset of an enterocele.
In two patients with only rectoceles we repeated defaecography after laxation because of other reasons. We now found:

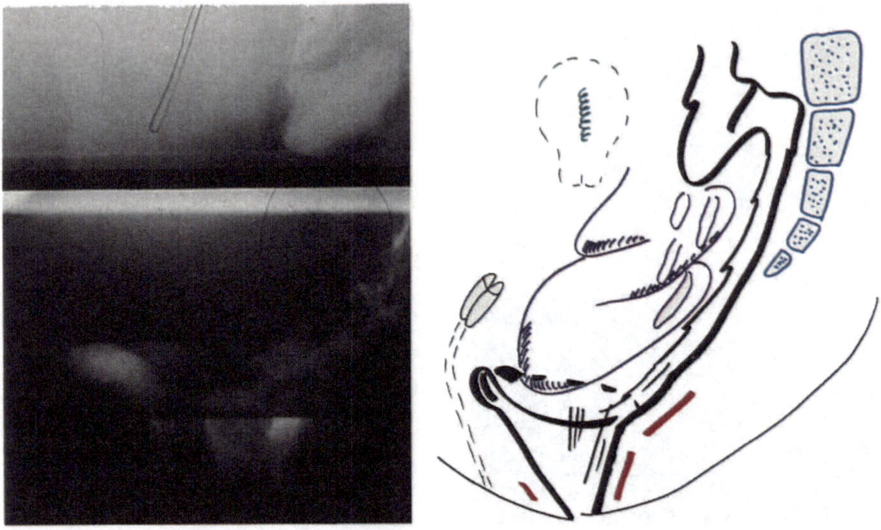

**Fig. 17.18.** Same patient as in Fig. 17.17. Large enterocele containing small intestine with opening of the anal canal (tendency towards rectal prolapse)

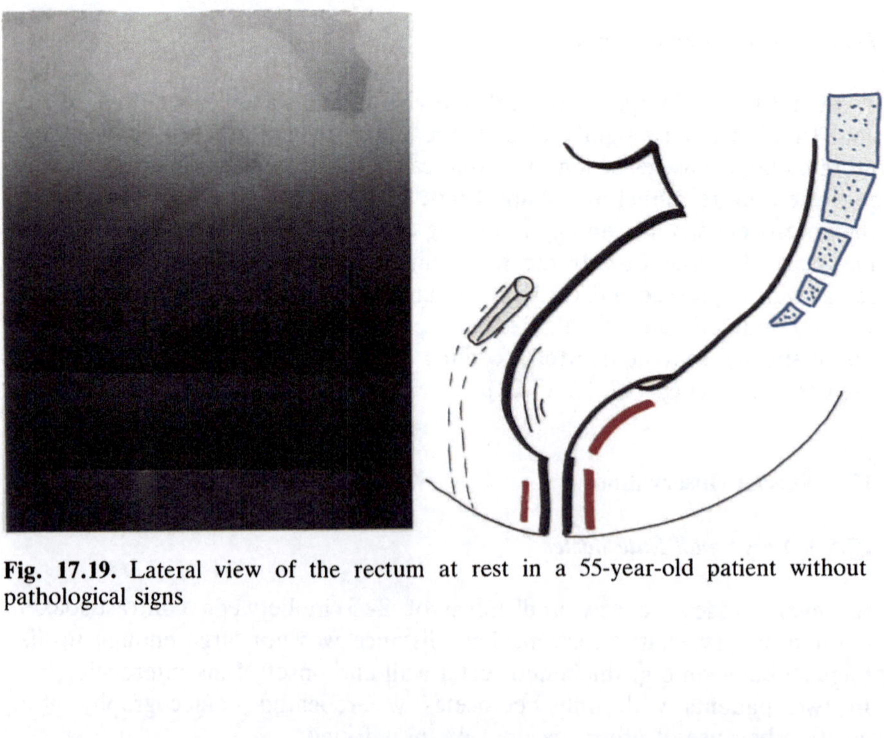

**Fig. 17.19.** Lateral view of the rectum at rest in a 55-year-old patient without pathological signs

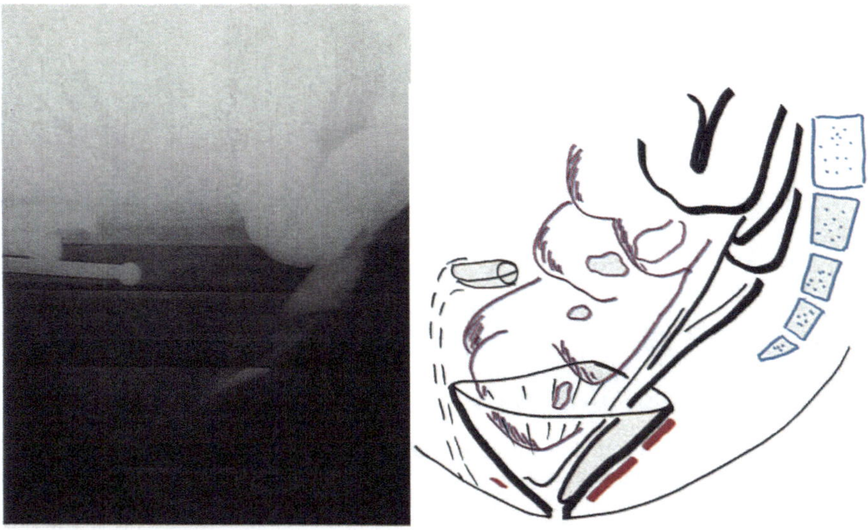

**Fig. 17.20.** Same patient as in Fig. 17.19. There is an eggcup-like deformation of the preanal rectum. The enterocele, containing large bowel, sits like an egg in an eggcup formed by rectum

- In one case the onset of a colon-filled enterocele (Figs. 17.1, 17.2, 17.23)
- In the other case, in which an IUD rendered the uterus visible, a small intestine-filled enterocele with an "egg-cup phenomenon" (Figs. 17.17, 17.18, 17.24)

### *17.5.2 Enteroceles and Hysterectomy*

In our experience enteroceles are very frequent after hysterectomy (Table 17.2). Impairment of the stability of the muscular pelvic floor is likely to occur in the case of extended, destroyed or infiltrated ligaments which can not be reconstructed by surgery.

The defaecographic appearance of an enterocele after hysterectomy normally does not differ greatly from that of an enterocele when the uterus is present.

If the ligaments of the "genital lamina" (see Chap. 3) cannot be retained and fixed during gynaecological or surgical intervention, e.g. in the case of extended hysterectomy the function of the genital lamina is destroyed. No enterocele can appear according to the employed definition because there is no hernial aperture with its lateral confinement, i.e. the uterosacral ligaments – a situation termed "*grande fosse pelvienne*" in the European literature.

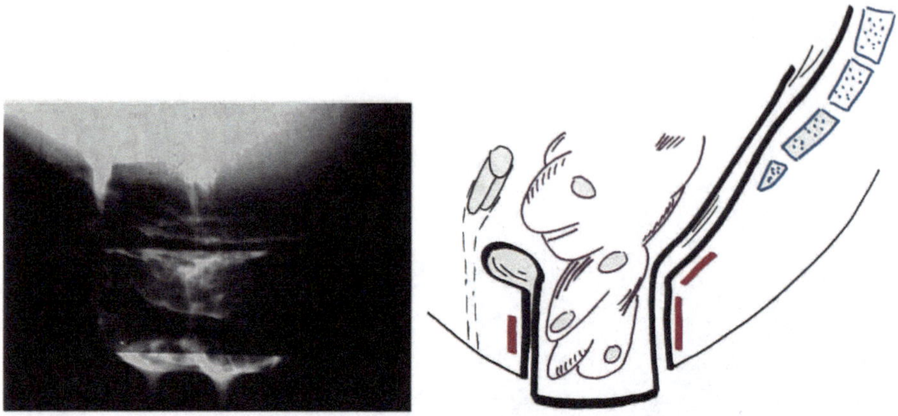

**Fig. 17.21.** 42-year-old female with very distended anal canal. In the lateral view, an enterocele containing small intestine (identified by air bubbles) is seen pressing the roof of the rectum throughout the anal canal. Remaining rectocele gives the appearance of a "doubled" anal canal

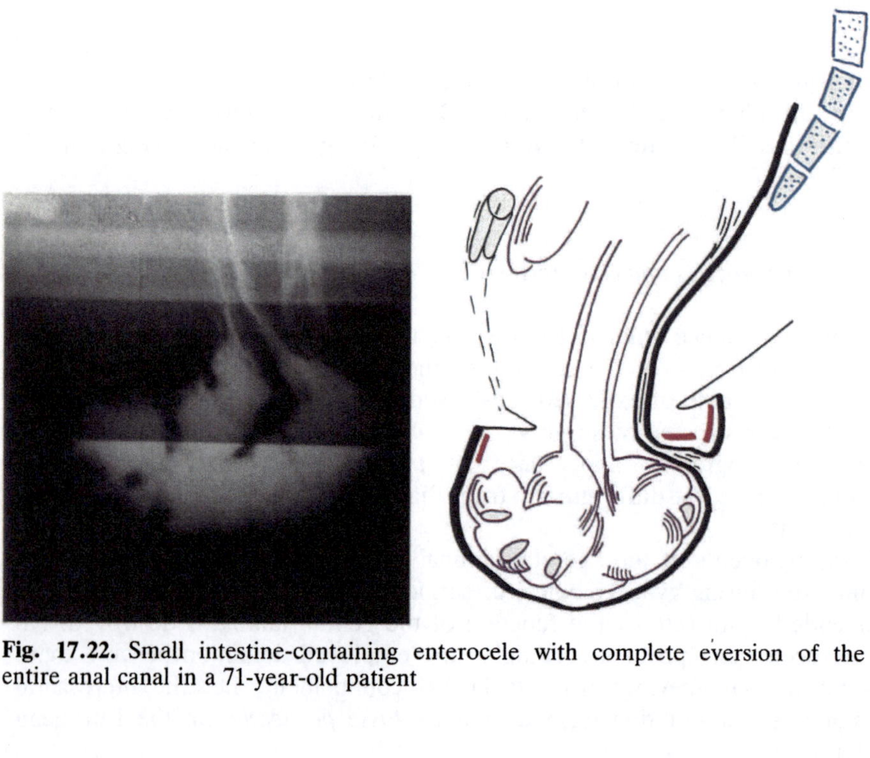

**Fig. 17.22.** Small intestine-containing enterocele with complete eversion of the entire anal canal in a 71-year-old patient

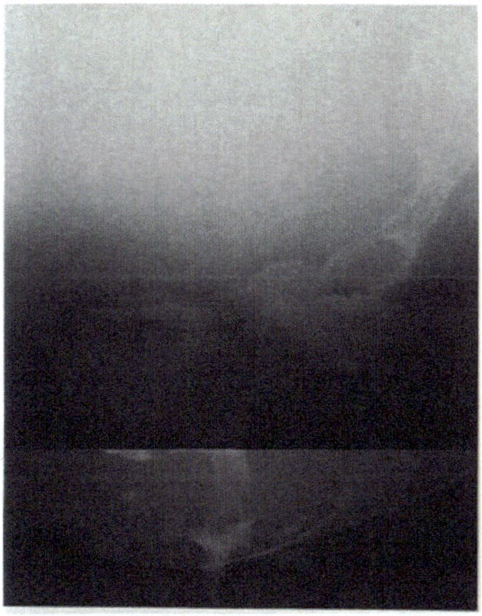
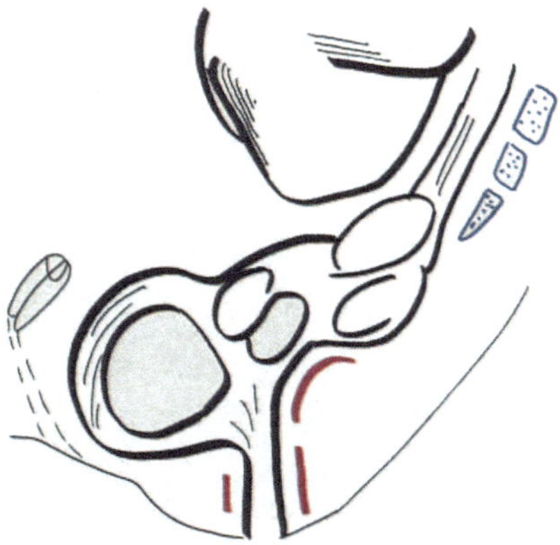

**Fig. 17.23.** Same patient as in Figs. 17.1 and 17.2. After a bulk diet no enterocele formation is observed

**Table 17.2.** Influence of hysterectomy on the frequency of enterocele (6.2.86–3.8.88: 473 female patients)

| | Enterocele | |
|---|---|---|
| | Yes | No |
| Hysterectomy | | |
| Yes | 33 | 62 |
| No | 88 | 290 |

Relationship significant at the $P \leqslant 0.025$ level.

Radiographs show that when intestinal pressure increases, a contrast-soaked tampon is pushed in a ventral direction, sliding on a filled or empty rectocele. In our illustrated case (Fig. 17.25) the vaginal tampon is on the top of the rectocele.

## 17.6 Conclusion

Using defaecography, enteroceles can be diagnosed even at an early stage. Small enteroceles may sometimes occur even under physiological conditions. Constant enteroceles can be defined as regards their form, location, content and relation to adjacent organs. The exact interpretation of radiographs

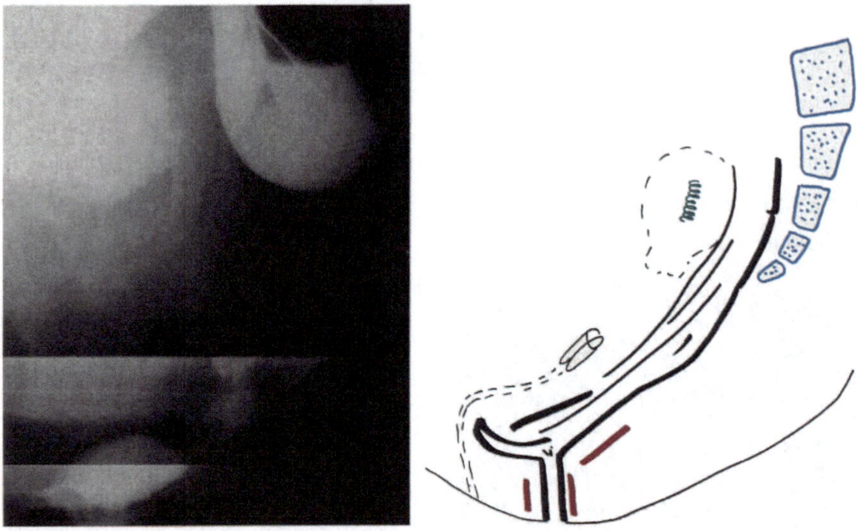

**Fig. 17.24.** Same patient as in Figs. 17.17 and 17.18. After a bulk diet the colon is filled. It presses the IUD-containing uterus against the rectum, thereby occluding the hernial aperture

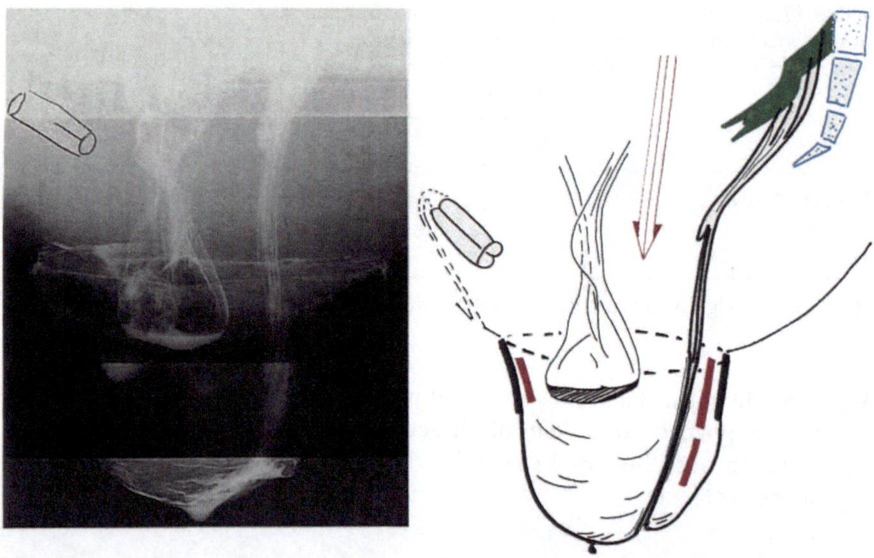

**Fig. 17.25.** During hysterectomy the uterine ligaments could not be reconstructed. Aspect of evacuated rectum shows complete rectal prolaps and enterocele grande fosse pelvienne in a 49-year-old patient

shows involvement of the muscular pelvic floor and any tendency towards rectal or vaginal prolapse. With better understanding of the disorders caused by enteroceles, gynaecologists and surgeons may find successful forms of treatment.

## References


1. Anthuber C, Obernitz N von, Denecke H (1989) Blood-outlet-Obstruction bei Rekto-Enterocele. Inzidenz, Diagnostik und postoperative Ergebnisse. Gynakol Rundsch 29 [Suppl 2]:59–60
2. Bartram CI, Turnball GK, Lennard-Jones JE (1988) Evacuation proctography: An investigation of rectal expulsion in 20 subjects without defecatory disturbance. Gastrointest Radiol 13:72–80
3. Beecham CI, Beecham JB (1973) Correction of prolapsed vagina or enterocele with fascia lata. Obstet Gynecol 42(4):542–546
4. Buchmann P (1988) Lehrbuch der Pathologie. Huber, Bern
5. Choi D, Ekberg O (1988) Functional analysis of anorectal junction: defecography. RÖFO 148(1):50–53
6. Cruikshank G (1987) Preventing posthysterectomy vaginal vault prolapse and enterocele during vaginal hysterectomy. Am J Obstet Gynecol 156(6):1433–1440
7. Doyle JF (1974) A case of spontaneous rupture of an enterocele following vaginal hysterectomy. J Ir Med Assoc 67(1):25–26
8. Geile D, Hauck R, Heilmann KL (1989) Der Deszensus des Beckenbodens – die häufigste proktologische Erkrankung? Endoskopie des Internisten, 9. Seminar Wiesbaden, 1–8
9. Geile D, Hauck R, Heilmann KL, Rath M, Ahrends W, Petery K (1988) Differentialdiagnose und Therapie innerer Prolapsformen in der Proktologie. Fortschr Gastroenterol Endosk 18
10. Gooley NA, Kuhnke M, Eusebio EB (1987) Acute transanal ileal evisceration. Dis Colon Rect 30(6):479–481
11. Guttman A, Afilalo M (1990) Vaginal evisceration. Am J Emerg Med 8(2):127–128
12. Hackle EJ, Parks T (1986) The pathogenesis and pathophysiology of rectal prolapse and solitary rectal ulcer syndrome. Clin Gastroenterol 15(4):985–1002
13. Haest JW, Broeders GH, Hoogeveen AJ (1979) Abdominal surgical treatment of enterocele. Eur J Obstet Gynecol Reprod Biol 7(1):55–56
14. Hauck R, Hauck-Schröder R (1988) Die Defäkographie in der Praxis. Annual Meeting der Bayerischen Röntgengesellschaft
15. Holland JB (1972) Enterocele and prolapse of the vaginal vault. Clin Obstet Gynecol 15(4):1145–1154
16. Jaisle F (1981) Die operative Behandlung der Enterocele und des Scheidenblindsackvorfalles. Geburtshilfe Frauenheilkd 41(11):777–780
17. Käser O, Ihlé FA (1960) Atlas der gynäkologischen Operationen. Thieme, Stuttgart
18. Lucente V, Benson JT (1990) Vaginal muellerian cyst presenting as an anterior enterocele: a case report. Obstet Gynecol 76(5 Pt 2):906–908
19. Mahieu P, Pringot J, Bodart P (1984) Defecography: II. Contribution to the diagnosis of defecation disorders. Gastrointest Radiol 9(3):253–261
20. Naessberger L (1984) Enterocele due to continuous ambulatory peritoneal dialysis (CARD). Acta Obstet Gynecol Scand 63(3):783
21. Nichols DH (1972) Types of enterocele and principles underlying choice of operation for repair. Obstet Gynecol 40(4):257–263

22. Ranney B (1981) Enterocele, vaginal prolapse, pelvic hernial recognition and treatment. Am J Obstet Gynecol 140(1):53–61
23. Richter K, Hausegger K, Lissner J, Kümper HJ, Koch J, Macketanz B (1974) Die Dochtmethode. Eine vervollkommnete Art der Kolpocystorectographie. Geburtshilfe Frauenheilkd 34:711–719
24. Schepens MA, Vanderveken MA, Gerard VE (1989) Herniation of the small intestine through an incised rectal prolapse. Case report. Acta Chir Scand 155(9):495–496
25. Shorvon PJ, McHugh S, Diamant NE, Somers S, Stevenson GW (1989) Defecography in normal volunteers: results and implications. Gut 30(12): 1737–1749
26. Svendsen JH, Galatius H, Hansen PK (1985) Spontaneous rupture of vaginal enterocele. Case report. Ann Chir Gynecol 74:43–45
27. Thiele H, Pampel R (1976) Scheidenruptur mit Dünndarmprolaps. Zentralbl Gynaekol 98(15):948–949
28. Webb MJ (1981) Enterocele: Prophylaxe und Therapie. Gynäkologe 14(3): 187–191
29. Zacharin RF (1980) Pulsion enterocele: review of functional anatomy of the pelvic floor. Obstet Gynecol 55(2):135–140
30. Zacharin RF, Hamilton NT (1972) The problem of the large enterocele. Aust N Z J Obstet Gynecol 12(2):105–109

# 18 Assessment of Functional Constipation

J.H.C. Kuijpers

Defaecation is considered to be the last taboo. People find it hard to talk about their defaecation habits. It is embarrassing and considered to be an indecent subject. On the other hand there is much folklore and mythology associated with the need for a daily evacuation, such as the belief that toxic substances may be absorbed into the body when a daily bowel movement does not occur. This is an obvious explanation for the huge amounts of laxatives that people use to treat themselves in order to have a daily bowel movement.

Constipation, however, is not a disease, but a symptom of many diseases of mixed origins and mechanisms. Description of complaints is difficult, as already mentioned. Most patients have vague, dull abdominal pain, cramps and fullness. They complain of nausea, a feeling of urge to defaecate and rectal obstruction, resulting in a need for straining. The perineum is often painful as a result. The incidence of digital defaecation is high, up to 30%. Patients frequently hesitate to admit it but subsequently state that it is done to initiate defaecation by opening the anal canal, to remove the impacted faeces from the rectum or to support the perineum during defaecation straining [1–3].

The aim in the treatment of chronic constipation is the restoration of a normal frequency and consistency of stool, and freedom from the discomforts ordinarily associated with constipation. The majority of affected patients have identifiable endocrine, metabolic or pharmacological reasons for their constipation, or can be easily managed with simple measures such as manipulation of diet, addition of bulk, regular exercises and careful use of laxatives and stool softeners. But when constipation persists despite dietary measures and no causative abnormalities are detected by conventional investigative procedures, further investigation is necessary.

Since colonic transit is a result of colonic function, constipation is a functional and not an anatomical disorder. It is therefore obvious that in studying, analysing and diagnosing functional constipation, conventional investigative procedures such as colonoscopy and barium enema are worthless since they only provide static data. Results of functional diagnostic tests are obligatory. If faecal continence is considered to be the ability to perceive, retain and excrete rectal filling, functional constipation is a continence disorder, or rather an excretion disorder which represents an indication for application of the colorectal laboratory.

## 18.1 The Colorectal Laboratory

The colorectal laboratory is a collection of dynamic tests that have been developed to study the function of the mechanism of continence, or rather, the colon, anorectum and pelvic floor muscle [4, 5]. In studying functional constipation, especially anal manometry, defaecography, electromyography and transit studies are of importance.

### *18.1.1 Anal Manometry*

Many different techniques have been advocated to measure anal canal pressures. Differences in technique are based on the location and the amount of catheter opening(s), types of perfusion, techniques of withdrawal and diameters of catheters (see also Chap. 14). All techniques have their own normal values. Resting pressures stand for internal anal sphincter function and squeeze pressures for external anal sphincter function. A decrease in resting pressure during inflation of a rectal balloon demonstrates internal anal sphincter relaxation, which excludes Hirschsprung's disease. Impaired squeeze pressures in constipated patients may lead to faecal incontinence, especially after colonic resections [5].

### *18.1.2 Defaecography*

A suitable technique for studying rectal evacuation is to fill the rectum with a radio-opaque contrast medium and then allow the patient to strain and excrete the contrast medium under radiological visualisation, a procedure named defaecography, cineradiography or cineproctography (see also Chaps. 5–8). It provides a picture of the successive phases of defaecation and may reveal disorders of defaecation. The anorectal angle, the intersection of the axes of the anal canal and rectum, is a measure of pelvic floor function. During defaecation straining the angle increases due to pelvic floor relaxation, while during squeezing it decreases as a result of muscle contraction [6].

### *18.1.3 Electromyography of the Pelvic Floor Muscle*

Electrical activity can be recorded by the non-invasive anal plug technique and invasively by putting a needle into the external and sphincter or

puborectalis muscle. Contraction and relaxation, but also denervation and reinnervation, can thus be recorded (see also Chap. 14).
The pelvic floor muscle is a rather unique muscle in that it shows some electrical activity at rest where other striated muscles are quiet, so that it can adequately and immediately react to an increase in abdominal pressure in order to maintain faecal continence.

### *18.1.4 Colonic Transit Time Studies*

The progression time of markers along the colon is an objective indication of colonic transit time (see also Chap. 13). They may be x-rayed in the stool or abdomen [7, 8]. Mean segmental transit time (right colon, left colon and rectosigmoid) can be calculated by giving a certain amount of markers (ten) over a certain number of days (five or ten), obtaining an abdominal radiograph on the next day (6th or 11th) and dividing it into zones corresponding to the right colon, left colon and rectosigmoid. From the numbers of markers present in each zone the mean segmental transit time can be calculated [9].
Several patterns of marker distribution can be recognised. Besides a normal transit through all three segments there is outlet obstruction (delayed transit through the rectosigmoid), hindgut dysfunction (delay through the left colonic and rectosigmoid segment) and slow colonic transit (delayed transit through all three segments). About 70%–80% of patients can be thus classified, but in about 20% there is an irregular and inconclusive pattern of distribution. An interesting and unexpected finding in several studies is that up to half of patients complaining of constipation have a normal total colonic transit time, indicating that constipation is not merely related to a low frequency of defaecation.

## 18.2 Types of Constipation

Two causes of functional constipation have been recognised in applying the colorectal laboratory. In the "functional outlet obstruction" type, transit through the abdominal colon is usually normal but rectal emptying is delayed due to a paradoxical contraction of the pelvic floor during defaecation straining which keeps the anal canal closed. In the "slow transit" type, colonic transit is delayed due to an impaired or dyscoordinated peristalsis; defaecation itself is normal.

### *18.2.1 Functional Outlet Obstruction*

Several authors have reported on the phenomenon that in some patients with constipation, barium could not be evacuated during defaecography or balloon proctography. No change in the anorectal angle on straining and no pelvic descent occurred. It was suggested that the muscle did not relax during straining, but remained contracted and prevented evacuation, thus causing a functional outlet obstruction [10–12]. Simultaneous recording of defaecography and electromyography of the pelvic floor in these patients demonstrated an abnormal increase in the activity of the puborectalis muscle and external anal sphincter during straining, associated with a failure to widen the anorectal angle. The simultaneously recorded anorectal pressure did not differ significantly from that in normals, which indicated that an adequate technique to increase intra-abdominal pressure was also used by the constipated patients. The radiological picture was therefore indeed caused by pelvic floor contraction. Furthermore, since anal manometry revealed normal resting and squeeze pressures, and internal sphincter inhibitory reflexes were present in all patients studied, it was concluded that this pelvic floor disorder was caused by an abnormal use of a normal muscle, rather than by an abnormal muscle.

Rectal evacuation studies tend to be unpleasant for the patient since they may lead to the embarrassment of passing flatus or even faeces during the tests in the presence of other people. The patient might therefore keep his muscle contracted to avoid this embarrassment, thus producing the abnormal radiological or electrical picture which has led investigators to believe that they have discovered a new functional disorder. So, since any person with a normal pelvic floor could demonstrate this radiological picture, the question arose as to whether the persistent contraction was due to the continuous action of an embarrassed patient occurring only during the investigation, or really represented a functional disorder of the pelvic floor causing outlet obstruction. A segmental colonic transit study was performed to investigate this question. The pattern of marker distribution that could be expected to prevail in the presence of such a functional disorder would be that of rectosigmoid delay. This pattern was indeed found in 60% [13, 14]. It was therefore concluded that the persistent contraction of the pelvic floor during defaecation straining does indeed represent a functional disorder of evacuation, for which the names the "spastic pelvic floor syndrome", "puborectalis syndrome", "non-relaxing pelvic floor" and "anismus" have been proposed.

Patients with the "spastic pelvic floor syndrome" contract their external anal sphincter when straining at defaecation, which closes off the anal canal and prevents evacuation. This causes faeces to accumulate in the rectum, leading to a severe and persistent urge to defaecate. They therefore strain heavily and persistently at stool, but these efforts are often in vain.

Paradoxical contraction of the pelvic floor has also been reported in patients with the "solitary rectal ulcer syndrome" and the "descending perineum syndrome" [15, 16]. Patients with a paradoxical contraction of the pelvic floor during straining can damage the anterior rectal wall by forcibly pressing it against, or even into, the closed anal canal during efforts to evacuate the rectum. Heavy and persistent straining at stool will lead not only to chronic ulceration of the rectal wall, but also to recurrent stretch injury of the pudendal and perineal nerves, resulting in impaired pelvic floor function and subsequent progressive perineal descent, the "descending perineum syndrome".

### *18.2.2 Slow Transit Constipation*

"Slow transit" constipation can be defined as a primary impairment of transport of faeces through the colon or part thereof. The diagnosis can be made when segmental transit times are prolonged and evacuation studies are normal. It is considered to be a neuromuscular disorder, classified as a disorder of the mesenteric plexus.

The colonic mesenteric plexus in these patients shows several abnormalities. The smooth muscle layers and mesenteric plexus appear normal and there are normal numbers of neurons within the plexus on H&E staining, but on silver staining there are reduced numbers of argyrophilic neurons and the remaining ones tend to be small and irregular, with uneven staining and fewer processes than normal. The ganglionic areas contain numerous, prominent, variably sized nuclei with active chromatin and faint cytoplasm. Axons are also decreased in number and there may be mild axonal degeneration and debris in some nerve tracts [17].

Some of these patients also have abnormal oesophageal peristalsis, delayed gastric emptying and a delayed small bowel transit [1]. The clinical syndrome caused by the enteric plexus abnormality is a result of loss of normal peristalsis and transport, the occurrence of spontaneous and uncoordinated contractions and loss of normal cyclical events such as the migrating motor complex.

## References


1. Kuijpers JHC (1990) Application of the colorectal laboratory in the diagnosis and treatment of functional constipation. Dis Colon Rectum 33:35–39
2. Devroede G (1983) Constipation: mechanisms and management. In: Sleisenger MH, Fordtran JS (eds) Gastrointestinal disease, pathophysiology, diagnosis and management, 3rd edn. Saunders, Philadelphia, pp 288–308
3. Constipation (1980) In: Goldberg SM, Gordon PH, Nivatvongs S (eds) Essentials of anorectal surgery. Lippincott, Philadelphia, pp 269–281

4. Kuijpers JHC (1988) Diagnosis and treatment of defecation disorders. Scand J Gastroenterol 23 [Suppl 154]:72–78
5. Smith LE (1990) Practical guide to anorectal testing. 1st edn. Ikagu-Shoin, New York
6. Mahieu P, Pringot J, Bodart P (1984) Defecography: 1. Description of a new procedure and results in normal patients. Gastrointest Radiol 9:247–251
7. Hinton JM, Lennard-Jones JE, Young AC (1969) A new method for studying gut transit times using radio-opaque markers. Gut 10:842–847
8. Arhan P, Devroede G, Jehannin B (1981) Segmental colonic transit time. Dis Colon Rectum 24:625–629
9. Metcalf AM, Phillips SF, Zinsheimer AR, MacCarty RL, Beart RW, Wolff BG (1987) Simplified assessment of segmental colonic transit. Gastroenterology 92:40–47
10. Kuijpers JHC, Bleijenberg G (1985) The spastic pelvic floor syndrome. A cause of constipation. Dis Colon Rectum 28:669–672
11. Preston DM, Lennard-Jones JE (1984) The balloon proctogram. Br J Surg 71:29–32
12. Womack NR, Williams NS, Holmfield JHM, Morrison JFB, Simkins KC (1985) New method for the dynamic assessment of anorectal function in constipation. Br J Surg 72:994–998
13. Jones PN, Lubowski DZ, Swash M, Henry MM (1987) Is paradoxical contraction of the puborectalis muscle of functional importance? Dis Colon Rectum 30:667–670
14. Kuijpers JHC, Bleijenberg G, DeMorree H (1986) The spastic pelvic floor syndrome; colonic outlet obstruction caused by pelvic floor disorder. Int J Colorect Dis 1:44–48
15. Rutter KPR (1974) Electromyographic changes in certain pelvic floor abnormalities. Proc R Soc Med 67:53–56
16. Kuijpers JHC, Schreve R, Ten Cate Hoedemakers H (1986) Diagnosis of disorders of continence causing the solitary rectal ulcer syndrome. Dis Colon Rectum 29:126–129
17. Krishnamurthy S, Schuffler MD (1987) Pathology of neuromuscular disorders of the small intestine and colon. Gastroenterology 93:610–639

# 19 Defaecography and Incontinence

M.-C. Marti

Incontinence can be defined as an inability to retain the rectal contents (solid or liquid faeces and gas) or to control excretion in inappropriate places or at inappropriate times. Incontinence is not caused by a single dysfunction or anomaly, but by several related disturbances interfering with the normal mechanisms of continence.

## 19.1 Mechanisms of Continence

Continence is achieved by several mechanisms [6]:

1. The flutter valve mechanism: puborectalis muscle contraction and posterior fixation of the lower rectum create an S-shaped double-binding of the anorectal junction with a translation of the anal axis in regard to the rectal axis.
2. The external sphincter, puborectalis sling and levator ani are responsible for voluntary continence and control of voiding. Voluntary contraction is time limited (less than 60 s) due to high muscular fatigability.
3. Rectal visco-elasticity, or rectal compliance. After 60 s of voluntary contraction of striated muscles, the anorectal reflex induces an increase in rectal compliance, allowing an increase in the rectal reservoir, a decrease in the rectal pressure and reduced stimulation of the striated muscles.
4. The permanent tone of the internal sphincter, which decreases only during bowel motion. Any destruction or excessive stretching of the internal sphincter results in a low resting tone with impaired control of liquids or gas.
5. Anal cushions ensure closing of the anal lumen. Their destruction or injury due to excessive excision reduces sensibility of the anal canal and interferes with continence.

Table 19.1 summarises the anatomical structures involved in maintaining continence.

**Table 19.1.** Anatomical structures maintaining continence

| |
|---|
| Rectum and rectal visco-elasticity |
| Flutter valve |
| Levator ani |
| Puborectalis sling |
| External sphincter |
| Internal sphincter |
| Anal cushions |

**Table 19.2.** Causes of faecal incontinence

| |
|---|
| Sensory problems |
| Destruction of sensory receptors |
| Continuous stimulation of sensory receptors |
| Muscular problems |
| Local lesions, distension |
| Tears and traumatic lesions |
| Degenerative lesions |
| Neurological problems |
| Neuropathy (diabetes) |
| Peripheral lesions (nervus pudendus internus) |
| Proximal lesions (spinal and caudal) |
| Psycho-organic problems |
| Alteration in rectal capacity and compliance |
| Destruction (low anterior resection, pull-through, sleeve anastomosis) |
| Alteration of visco-elastic properties (severe inflammatory lesions) |
| Prolapse, intussusception and rectoceles |

## 19.2 Mechanisms of Incontinence

Destruction or impaired function of any of the aforementioned mechanisms, singly or in association, may result in more or less severe incontinence. The various causes of incontinence are listed in Table 19.2.

## 19.3 Severity of Incontinence

Pressure at rest or during straining can be correlated to some extent with incontinence: most patients suffering from incontinence will have low pressures. Nevertheless, normal subjects may have low pressures and incontinent patients, high pressures. Severity of incontinence is in fact far better assessed according to the nature of incontinence (solid stools, liquids or flatus) and the frequency of incontinence episodes (several times a week, from once a month to once a week, less than once a month). A score (Table 19.3) may be calculated ranging from perfect continence (score 0) to complete incontinence (score 18).

**Table 19.3.** Incontinence score

| Degree | Frequency | Flatus | Liquids | Solids |
|---|---|---|---|---|
| I | Less than 1 x/month | 1 | 4 | 7 |
| II | 1 x/month to 1 x/week | 2 | 5 | 8 |
| III | More than 1 x/week | 3 | 6 | 9 |

## 19.4 Investigations in Cases of Incontinence

The diagnosis of incontinence is achieved by reference to medical history records and by clinical examinations, as described in Chap. 4. The particular procedures useful for investigating incontinence are as follows [6]:

*Manometry.* By means of manometry performed with balloon, open-tipped catheters or micro-transducers, one can collect data on anal pressure at rest and during straining, and on anal length by establishing a pressure profile. Data can be collected before and after treatment in order to evaluate functional results. The recto-anal reflex can be elicited to evaluate the integrity of the spinal reflexes.

*EMG.* For establishing neuropathy, EMG, and especially single-fibre EMG, is the investigative method of choice. Furthermore, with EMG, mapping of a sphincter defect is possible.

*Pudendal Nerve Latency.* Delay between stimulation of the pudendal nerve and registration of sphincter activity is called pudendal nerve latency. In the presence of neuropathy, this delay is prolonged, while in the presence of myopathy the latency is unchanged.

*Volumetry.* One may perform volumetry of the rectum either by means of perfusion of the rectum or with a distended balloon. It is possible to determine the minimum volume perceived by the patient the volume producing pain, and the volume inducing uncontrolled voiding. If pressure within the balloon is simultaneously measured and correlated to the volume of the rectum, visco-elasticity of the reservoir can be calculated.

*Sphincteric Resistance.* A 2-cm metal ball is introduced into the rectum. The strength required to expel the ball can be measured at rest and when the patient squeezes.

*Anal Sensibility.* Thermic changes and electrical stimulation within the anal canal yield information on the sensibility of the mucosa.

*Defaecography*. As an investigative method, defaecography is of very limited value in patients suffering from incontinence as they are unable to prevent leakage of barium [2–5]. Loss of contrast medium while filling the rectosigmoid with barium paste or when moving the patient can occur even with fully continent patients and may be due to the fluidity of the contrast medium or overdistension of the rectum. This should not be interpreted as incontinence.
Gross anatomical abnormalities associated with incontinence are clinically evident and do not have to be confirmed by radiological investigations. Functional neuromuscular abnormalities cannot be investigated by defaecography and require more sophisticated laboratory investigations to assess their precise cause.

## 19.5 Quantitative Values

In patients suffering from incontinence, several abnormalities are noticeable on defaecography [4, 5, 7]:

- *Reduced translation* of anal axis to rectal axis: The distance between the anal canal axis and the rectal axis normally represents 60% of the pubococcygeal distance. Any reduction of this proportion may result in gross faecal incontinence (Fig. 19.1).
- *Increased anorectal angle* at rest is the most common anomaly observed in cases of incontinence. Mahieu and co-workers [2, 3] found that an anorectal posterior angle exceeding 130° invariably revealed incontinence. There is no correlation between the anorectal angle and maximal basal pressure, maximal squeeze pressure, maximal contraction pattern and moment of first leak [1].

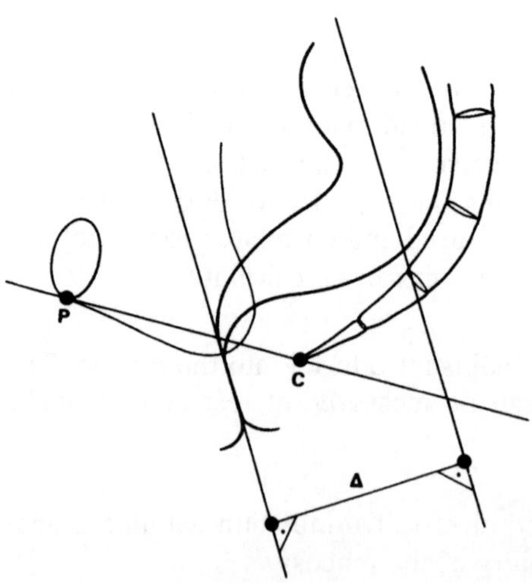


**Fig. 19.1.** Translation of anal canal axis and rectal axis. Δ = 60% of *CP* (pubococcygeal distance) in continent patients

- *A wide upper anal canal* may be related to a diminished tone of the upper part of the internal sphincter. This may result in urgency even if the squeeze pressure of the external sphincter and puborectalis sling is high. A wide upper anal canal may be associated with intussusception of the anterior rectal wall and with a persistent fingerprint of the puborectalis on lateral films, even during straining. This does not mean that the puborectalis does not relax and that the patient suffers from anismus. It may just reflect a compensatory hypertrophy of the puborectalis sling in order to improve continence and to correct a weak central perineum.
- *Limited Compliance of the Rectum*. It is possible to measure the volume of contrast medium necessary to fill the rectum. Sclerosis and/or chronic inflammation of the rectal wall may reduce rectal volume and compliance and result in urgency and repeated evacuation.
- *Descending perineum*. Descent of the tip of the anorectal angle can be measured on lateral films during defaecography and with the use of a St. Mark's perineometer. At rest, during straining and while squeezing, the angle's position can be compared with the pubococcygeal line, to the top of the femoral head and the lower part of the ischium. Any excessive increase in the descent (more than 5 cm) is an indirect sign of pudendal neuropathy, frequently associated with incontinence.

## 19.6 Associated Lesions

Incontinence may be associated with particular radiological pictures easy to detect on defaecography films.

### *19.6.1 Mucosal Prolapse and Intussusception*

Both mucosal prolapse and intussusception may result in faecal soiling; if the extremity of the mucosal fold at rest comes into contact with the upper part of the anal canal, mimicking a recto-anal reflex, reduced pressure of the upper part of the internal sphincter may occur, causing partial incontinence.

### *19.6.2 Solitary Rectal Ulcer*

Mucosal prolapse may result in a solitary rectal ulcer if the tone of the puborectalis sling increases to compensate for the reduced tone of the internal sphincter. This pathogenic mechanism can be proved by manometry coupled with EMG of the puborectalis sling and of the external sphincter.

### *19.6.3 Prolapse*

Incontinence is frequently associated with a rectal prolapse. In such situations, incontinence may be due to repeated or permanent overstretching of the sphincteric structures. In the presence of a descending perineum, incontinence (or "idiopathic" incontinence) and prolapse are often caused by pudendal neuropathy.

### *19.6.4 Rectocele*

Association of rectocele with incontinence is frequent and unfortunately underestimated. A rectocele is a hernia of the anterior rectal wall caused by a weak rectovaginal septum. The weakness may be due to obstetric injuries or overstretching while straining in the case of chronic constipation. While a rectocele may be caused by chronic straining, it may also result in outlet obstruction. In postmenopausal women, the trophicity of the rectovaginal septum is reduced.

Rectocele, whether asymptomatic or associated with constipation, may progressively be complicated by incontinence. Patients complain of a "roll-down" syndrome, incomplete evacuation, two-stage evacuation and even gross incontinence. The central part of the rectovaginal septum is lower than normal even in the absence of a descending perineum.

Digital examination shows a normotonic anal canal and good contraction of the puborectalis sling, but a short anterior anal canal. During examination, if the finger is introduced as far as the upper part of the puborectalis sling and is then rotated 180° clockwise at the same level, the fingertip is within the rectocele (Fig. 19.2). If the patient is asked to squeeze, a gap appears between the anterior anal canal and the puborectalis muscle, resulting in evacuation of the content of the lower part of the rectocele. This gap can be easily demonstrated digitally and is responsible for incontinence associated with rectocele (Fig. 19.3).

Defaecography confirms this particular mechanism of incontinence associated with rectocele. Films can show a short anterior anal canal, a rectocele, an intussusception or an anterosuperior mucosal fold, or a long posterior anal canal with a strong print of the puborectalis muscle. When squeezing, the puborectalis muscle does not close the anal canal but squeezes the rectocele and expels its content. Each retention effort results in a paradoxical evacuation of faeces or incontinence (Fig. 19.4).

**Fig. 19.4a–e.** Defaecography in a 72-year-old woman with rectocele and ▶ incontinence: **a** at rest; **b**, **c** development of rectocele while straining; **d**, **e** emptying of rectocele while squeezing. The anterior anal canal is shorter than the posterior anal canal

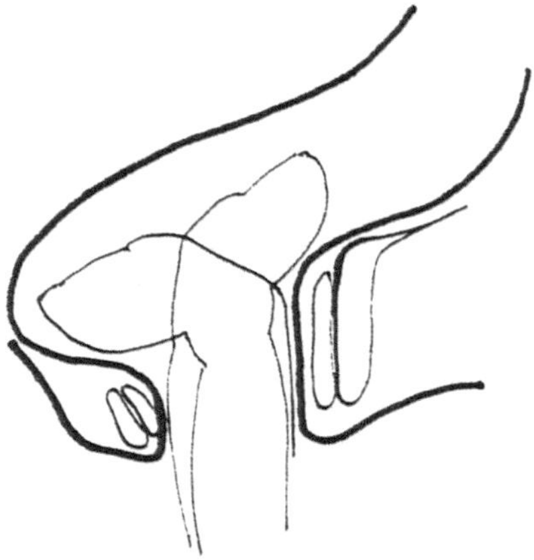

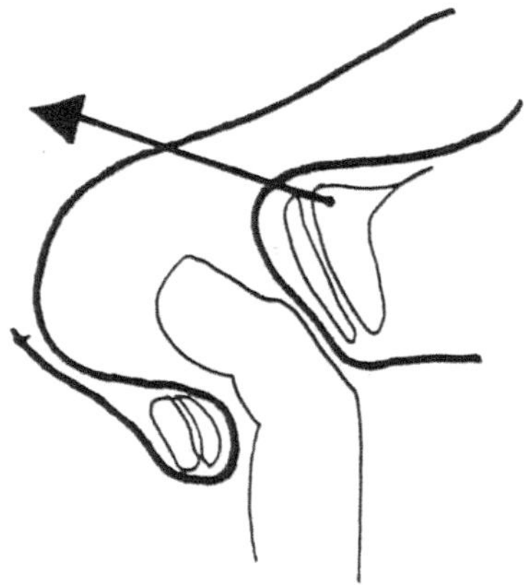

**Fig. 19.2** (*left*). Digital examination with the fingertip of the upper part of the puborectalis sling and, when rotated at the same level, of the rectocele. A short anterior anal canal is present

**Fig. 19.3** (*right*). Short anterior anal canal in a patient with rectocele. A gap appears when the patient squeezes

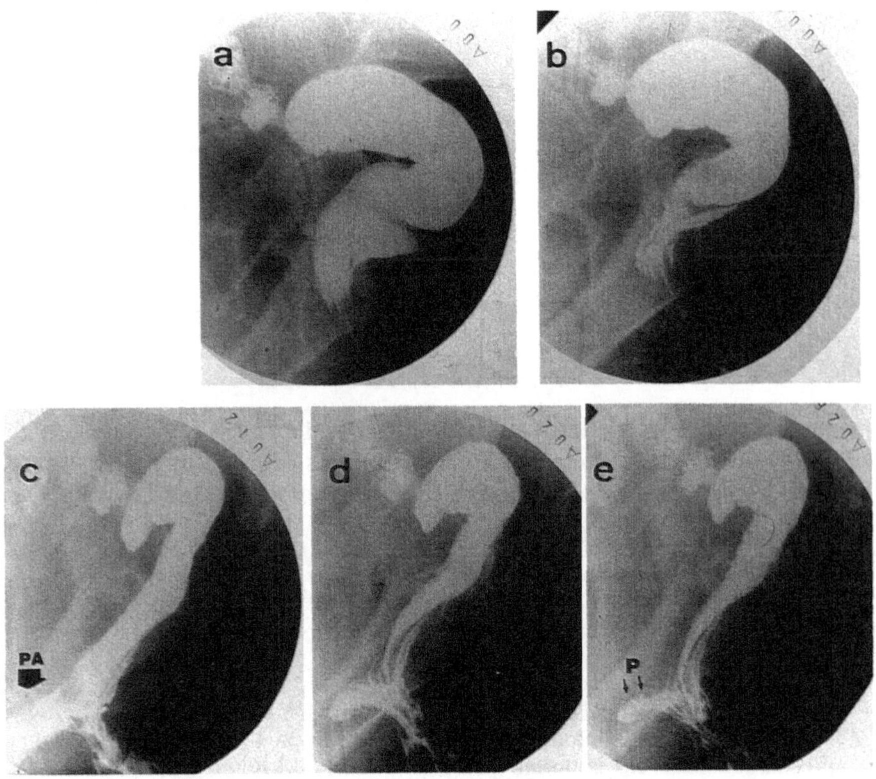

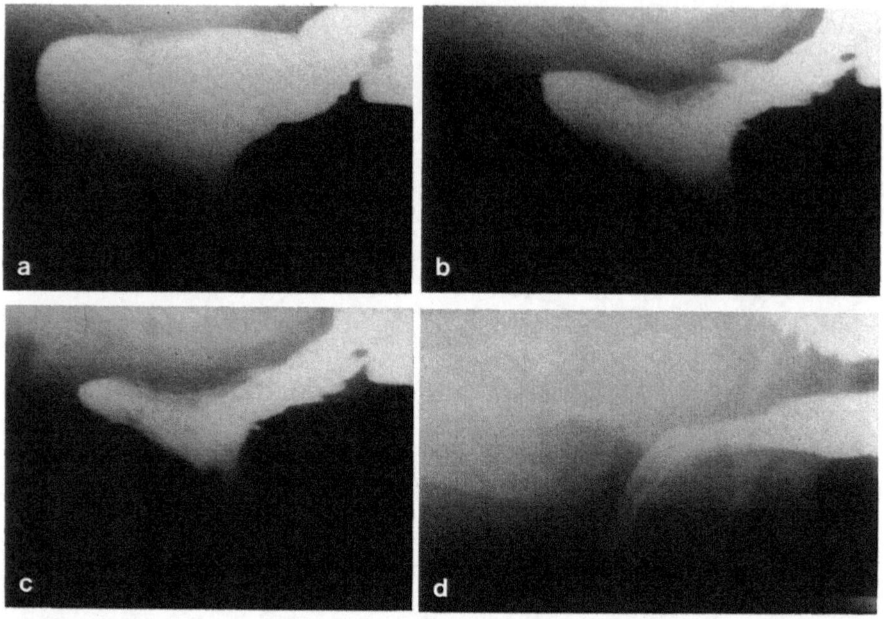


**Fig. 19.5a–d.** Defaecography in a 54-year-old woman. **a–c** Asymmetry of anal canal with incontinence and rectocele. **d** Postoperative state with correction of anal canal length

Digital examination and defaecography confirm the diagnosis, which may be suspected on the basis of precise clinical records.
Surgical treatment is successful: an endo-anal repair is performed, with longitudinal and transverse plication to lengthen the anterior part of the internal sphincter (Fig. 19.5).

## 19.7 Conclusion

Defaecography is of limited value in assessing the cause of severe, usually clinically evident, incontinence. For minor forms of incontinence, however, defaecography can be useful in demonstrating associated lesions which can be surgically corrected.

## References

1. Felt-Bersma RJF, Luth WJ, Janssen JJWM, Meuwissen SGM (1990) Defecography in patients with anorectal disorders. Dis Colon Rectum 33:277–284
2. Mahieu P, Pringet J, Bodart P (1984) Defecography I: description of a new procedure and results in normal patients. Gastrointest Radiol 9:247–251

3. Mahieu P, Pringet J, Bodart P (1984) Defecography II: contribution to the diagnosis of defecation disorders. Gastroentest Radiol 9:253–261
4. Marti M-C, Mirescu D (1982) Utilité du défécogramme en proctologie. Ann Gastroenterol Hepatol (Paris) 18:379–384
5. Marti M-C (1991) Défécographie ou rectographie dynamique. Ann Gastroenterol Hepatol (Paris) 27:109–112
6. Marti M-C (1991) Incontinence. In: Marti M-C, Givel J-C (eds) Surgery of anorectal diseases. Springer, Berlin Heidelberg New York, pp 205–217
7. Mirescu D, Sadry F (1991) Radiological investigation. In: Marti M-C, Givel J-C (eds) Surgery of anorectal diseases. Springer, Berlin Heidelberg New York, pp 34–45

# 20 Anal Sphincter Dysplasia

J. Hirsig

## 20.1 Introduction

Anal sphincter dysplasia (ASDP) was first described by Upadhyaya [1]. He published his intraoperative observations of the malformation of the superficial anal sphincter in seven children with an anterior perineal anus. Preceding Upadhyaya, Hendren [2] and Leap and Ramenofsky [3] had published their work on the relationship between childhood constipation and the anterior position of the anus.
The connection between constipation and an anteriorly displaced anus is described in many paediatric textbooks. In an early international classification of anorectal malformation [4] the anteriorly displaced anus was listed as the mildest form. In the most recent international classification [5] the anteriorly displaced anus was omitted because of the lack of evidence to substantiate that it is a true anatomical defect.
In 1985 I saw adult twin females with severe constipation and an extremely anteriorly located anus. Since then, I have seen a great number of adults suffering from a variety of defaecation disorders starting in childhood. All showed clinical findings comparable to those described by Hendren, such as an anteriorly displaced anus, a posterior shelf in the lower anal canal and a thin perineal body. In the beginning we treated these patients surgically with a modified Upadhyaya's procedure, which consisted manly of a butterfly-shaped anoplasty. Unfortunately, however, we observed recurrent constipation in many cases after a few months.
Since we were convinced that there must be an as yet unrecognised anatomical defect responsible for defaecation disorders starting in childhood, we began to study this problem with CT scanning of the pelvic floor and defaecography. We also had the opportunity to examine a great number of patients with early childhood onset constipation and study their pelvic floor anatomy intraoperatively. Because our operative technique had to be changed several times and our understanding of the anatomical problems is still far from clear, it is not possible to summarise our thoughts conclusively at the present time. But in view of the very encouraging operative results, a brief description of our theory will be given. It is important to realise that the following still has a very preliminary character. The aim of this publication is to draw the reader's attention to some new thoughts about anal function and its implications for the physiology of the gastrointestinal tract.

**Table 20.1.** Distribution of symptoms according to age in males ($n$ = 25)

| Symptoms | Age (years) | | |
|---|---|---|---|
| | 0–5 | 6–14 | 14–67 |
| Difficulties in evacuation | 6 | | |
| Difficulties in holding back | 10 | 5 | 2 |
| Global defaecation disorders | | | 2 |
| Total | 16 | 5 | 4 |

**Table 20.2.** Distribution of symptoms according to age in females ($n$ = 66)

| Symptoms | Age (years) | | |
|---|---|---|---|
| | 0–5 | 6–14 | 14–61 |
| Difficulties in evacuation | 3 | 3 | 37 |
| Difficulties in holding back | 5 | 4 | |
| Global defaecation disorders | 12 | | 2 |
| Total | 20 | 7 | 39 |

## 20.2 Symptoms

The symptoms we encountered in our patients cover the whole spectrum of complaints one encounters in proctology: difficulties in evacuation of hard stools (constipation), pain, anal bleeding, diarrhoea (often "paradoxical diarrhoea") and difficulties in holding back faecal evacuation (encopresis). Often constipation and encopresis alternate in the same patient, and we call this the "global defaecation disorder". The distribution of these complaints in a subgroup of our patients (n = 91) is summarised by age and sex in Tables 20.1 and 20.2.

It is quite logical that in small children global defaecation disorders are much more common than "classical" constipation with difficulties in evacuation of stools. Most of the parents report most peculiar defaecation patterns. Usually the children refuse the potty and then hide and evacuate their enormously large stools in their nappies. The procedure can sometimes take hours or even a whole day. Bleeding does not seem to worry the parents, because it is regularly delineated only after one asks about this symptom. The majority of the children had either been seen by a psychiatrist or the family had at least considered family therapy with a paediatric psychologist. If parents complain "only" about constipation one should ask about the defaecation pattern described above. Often they hesitate to tell the doctor about this grotesque behaviour.

According to the psychiatric literature, this behaviour is restricted to children and is not known in adults. We consider it, therefore, most interesting that among our 91 patients four adults (two men and two women) were referred because of problems with stool continence. In all four cases massive coprostasis was demonstrated as being responsible for faecal overflow.
We had the opportunity to question the parents of some of the adult women, about their daughters' defaecation patterns in early childhood. Many confirmed our hypothesis that at least some severely constipated adults had global defaecation disorders in early infancy. At the moment a survey is being done together with a psychiatrist to study the long-term results of psychotherapy in children with encopresis.
In ASDP, then, the whole defaecation event is impaired, the holding back and the evacuation.

## 20.3 Etiology

A genetic study carried out on 42 of our patients [6] revealed autosomal dominant inheritance with variable expression and probably incomplete penetrance of the mutated gene.

## 20.4 Clinical Signs

The clinical findings are difficult to describe. As Hendren noted, the anterior location of the anus is not always relevant. In most cases the dentate line reaches down to the anal verge, and the short ectodermal anal canal is responsible for the impaired anal sensation. A posterior shelf in the anal canal can not always be palpated, but if present this finding is diagnostic.

## 20.5 Anatomy

In spite of the lack of clear proof we think that the main pathogenic factor is the incomplete posterior fixation of the anal sphincter complex to the coccyx. In animals with a tail one can easily observe how the anus is pulled open by sphincter muscles extending to the tail. When humans lost the tail during evolution the posterior relationship of the sphincter muscle and the coccyx became a weak point.
Especially interesting, therefore, are patients with sacral agenesis. Usually it is thought that patients lacking more than three sacral elements invariably have neurogenic disorders of the rectum and bladder. This is certainly not true. Our three patients operated on for global defaecation disorders with

partial agenesis of the sacrum have regained full anorectal function after the posterior fixation of the sphincter complex.
We are therefore convinced that an appropriate dorsal fixation of the sphincter is essential for normal anal function. Whether this can be demonstrated conclusively on CT scans remains to be established.
In our experience CT or MRI of the pelvic floor cannot be omitted, especially since a presacral mass, regularly found in Curarino's triad, should be excluded prior to an operation. This association of anorectal, sacral and presacral anomalies, first described by Currarino et al. [7], is not as rare as one assumes. In our series of approximately 150 patients with severe defaecation disorders, this triad was diagnosed nine times by CT or MRI.

## 20.6 Technique and Outcome

Originally, as mentioned above, we used Upadhyaya's technique, but unfortunately most patients had recurrent problems after a few months. We then added fixation of the superficial anal sphincter to the coccyx. Now we believe that often the intervention must be more extensive. If necessary the whole pelvic floor has to be elevated, and sometimes the reconstruction of a malformed sphincter is required. Rectopexy should be done if there is any sign of rectal prolapse. But still the main aim is to achieve adequate dorsal fixation of the sphincter complex.
The results are very encouraging indeed. In almost all of the children operated on for ASDP, defaecation normalised within one year. In adults the results are not as good; this is due to the fact that after many years of intestinal stasis the function may irreversibly deteriorate. This condition may be compared to obstructive uropathy and could therefore be called "obstructive enteropathy". Contrary to what we had seen after Upadhyaya's operation, the later the follow-up the better the results after dorsal fixation of the sphincter complex in patients with ASDP.

## 20.7 Summary and Conclusion

Anal sphincter dysplasia is a congenital dysplasia and malfixation of the sphincter complex leading to severe sphincter dysfunction. Surgical repair before "irreversible" enteropathy has become established may improve the quality of life in patients with early childhood onset defaecation disorders.

## References

1. Upadhyaya P (1985) Mid – anal sphincter malformation, cause of constipation in anterior perineal anus. J Pediatr Surg 19:183–186
2. Hendren H (1978) Constipation caused by anterior location of the anus and its surgical correction. J Pediatr Surg 13:505–512
3. Leap LL, Ramenofsky ML (1978) Anterior ectopic anus. A common cause of constipation in children. J Pediatr Surg 13:627–630
4. Stephens FD, Durham-Smith E (1971) Anorectal malformations in children. Year Book Medical, p 133
5. Stephens FD, Durham-Smith E (1986) Classification, identification and assessment of surgical treatment of anorectal anomalies. Pediatr Surg 1:200–205
6. Zorzi A, Schinzel A, Hirsig J (1991) Analsphinkterdysplasie als Ursache chronischer Defäkationsstörungen: eine klinische und genetische Studie. Schweiz Med Wochenschr 121:1567–1575
7. Currarino G, Cold D, Votteler T (1981) Triad of anorectal, sacral and pre-sacral anomalies. Am J Roentgenol 137:395–398

# Subject Index

GPSR Compliance

*The European Union's (EU) General Product Safety Regulation (GPSR) is a set of rules that requires consumer products to be safe and our obligations to ensure this.*

*If you have any concerns about our products, you can contact us on ProductSafety@springernature.com*

In case Publisher is established outside the EU, the EU authorized representative is:

Springer Nature Customer Service Center GmbH
Europaplatz 3
69115 Heidelberg, Germany

**Batch number: 10620141**

Printed by Printforce, the Netherlands